The Radiology Report

A Guide to Thoughtful Communication
for Radiologists and Other Medical Professionals

Curtis P. Langlotz, MD, PhD

For Mary

Table of Contents

Chapter 1:
Perfect Pictures, Imperfect Prose

On a spring day in 1896, a standing-room-only crowd gathered at the New York Academy of Medicine to hear a lecture by Dr. William J. Morton. After paying tribute to Edison and Tesla, Dr. Morton embarked on a series of demonstrations that awed the crowd. He allowed over 100 audience members to view fluoroscopy of their own hands. Among other oddities, they clearly saw a healed finger fracture and a needle embedded in a woman's palm. A witty reporter described the best fluoroscopic views of the evening as "a trout, a flounder, and Dr. Morton's left foot in a boot."[1]

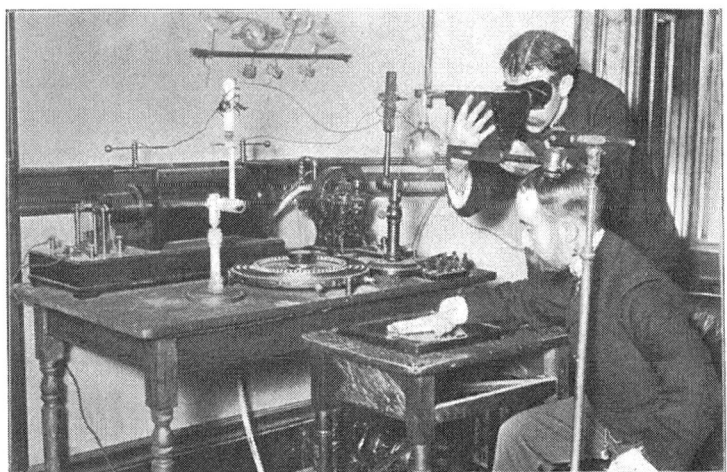

Figure 1. Dr. Morton conducting an experiment with Edwin Hammer, an electrical engineer. Figure 54 from reference [2].

Dr. Morton had studied the work of Dr. Wilhelm Roentgen and at the time was widely regarded as the foremost U.S. expert on the x-ray.[2] Just a few weeks later, he composed a handwritten letter to his colleague Dr. Leopold Stieglitz, a Park Avenue physician. His letter, shown in Figure 2, is one of the earliest known examples of a radiology report.[3,4]

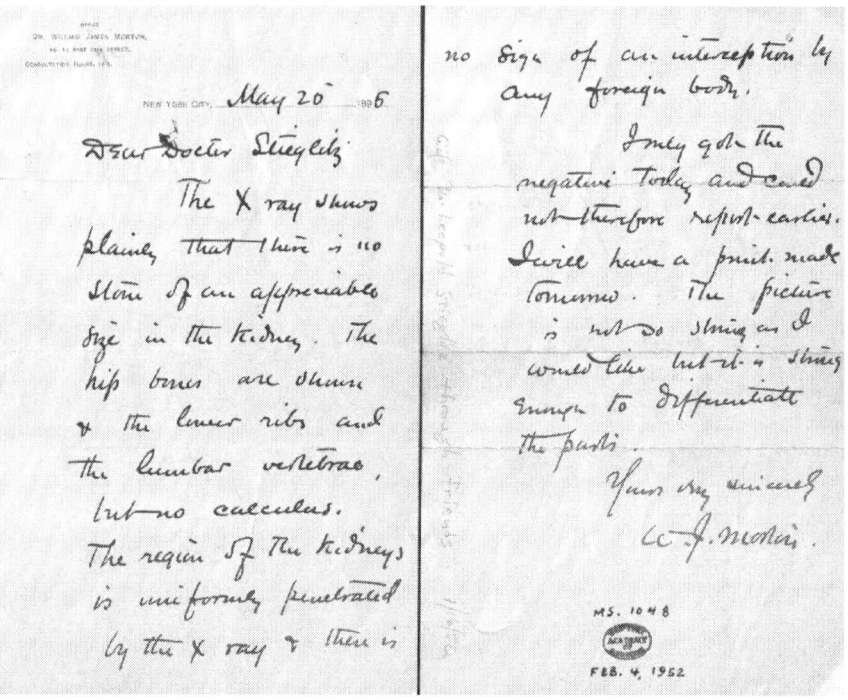

Dear Doctor Stieglitz,

The X ray shows plainly that there is no stone of an appreciable size in the kidney. The hip bones are shown and the lower ribs and the lumbar vertebrae, but no calculus. The region of the kidneys is uniformly penetrated by the X ray & there is no sign of an interception by any foreign body.

I only got the negative today and could not therefore report earlier. I will have a print made tomorrow. The picture is not so strong as I would like but it is strong enough to differentiate the parts.

Yours very sincerely,

W. J. Morton

Figure 2. One of the earliest known radiology reports.[3,4] (Courtesy of the New York Academy of Medicine Library.)

The Earliest Radiology Reports

The radiology report began as a letter between colleagues, describing what the images showed—analogous to reports from other clinical subspecialty consultations and strikingly similar to the narrative format we see today. These "reports" first became commonplace in the early 20th century, as radiography facilities began to proliferate in U.S. hospitals.

Anyone familiar with the pitfalls of modern radiology practice will note familiar elements of Dr. Morton's practice. Work flow issues ("I only got the negative today and could not therefore report earlier") and hedging related to image quality ("The picture is not so strong as I would like...") had early origins. Another harbinger of things to come: Dr. Morton's fee for a simple radiograph was $5 at a time when a hospital admission cost $1 per day and a physician house call cost $2.[3]

Radiology Communication a Century Later

...in order to make our reports more valuable they should be written in a manner ... that would convey distinct ideas as to the conditions present.
—Preston Hickey[5]

Nearly 100 years later, during my first rotation as a radiology resident, an attending radiologist quietly took me aside to a corner of the reading room. Under the dim light from a view box, we huddled over a small shelf as he covered one of my reports with red editor's marks. Kindly but firmly, he described the problems: Some passages were redundant; others were jumbled and ungrammatical; many were vague. Not a line went unscathed.

At the time, I bristled at the critique. But later, I came to appreciate the time he had taken to make me a better radiologist. I expected such constructive moments to be repeated throughout my training, transforming and optimizing my reporting methods as I became a more experienced trainee. But to my surprise, the only further feedback I received was the occasional barked complaint about a misspelling or a gross grammatical error.

Since that time, radiology training has improved: Many programs provide some didactic instruction on radiology reporting,[6] and some even provide regular constructive feedback on specific reports.[7–10] Several useful guides to radiology reporting have been published.[11–15] But a vast gap remains between the importance of radiology communication and the resources available to guide it.[16] At the end of the 20th century, 98% of residents received no

15

formal radiology reporting instruction. Instead, radiologists learn by apprenticeship and by "osmosis"—eavesdropping on their peers.[17]

Radiologists in training start from a low base: Most medical students have never dictated clinical documentation. And the learning curve is steep: Even experienced scientific writers are challenged by the radiology report because of its specific stylistic rules and unique organizational constraints. The lack of authoritative resources and regular reinforcement, together with the need for reporting speed, can prevent good reporting practices from taking hold. Thus, bad habits develop quickly, with an inevitable retention of the reporting patterns radiologists have followed for over a century: Describe what you see, with little forethought about the structure and function of the report.

The lack of resources and training shows itself in the quality of radiology reports.[18] Although the radiology report is arguably our most important work product, we create reports today in a haphazard way and produce a narrative that varies widely in character and quality. In one study of chest x-ray reports, 14 different terms were used to describe interstitial edema, and 23 words were used to suggest the presence of a finding.[19] Thirty-nine percent of referring providers are occasionally confused by imaging reports.[20] Fifty-one percent of referring physicians indicated that chest x-ray reports sometimes did not address the clinical question.[20] A multi-institutional study showed that 11% of chest x-ray reports for patients admitted for pneumonia failed to mention the presence or absence of pneumonia.[19] Studies continue to show that referring clinicians see the need for improvement.[20–25] Almost half a billion radiology reports were dictated last year, some inevitably resulting in missed follow-up, delayed diagnosis, and in some cases, malpractice claims.

A more insidious effect of our haphazard reporting methods is the inability to reuse information in radiology reports for performance improvement, practice management, and research. A decade after I encountered the red pen in the reading room, I received a similar wake-up call in the research laboratory. MR imaging was in its early heyday, and researchers were looking for data to prove its value. I led a team examining the relationship between prostate MR imaging and the likelihood of cancer recurrence, as measured by increases in serum prostate-specific antigen (PSA).[26] Unfortunately, we found that most of the prostate MR imaging reports were at best ambiguous and at worst internally inconsistent. In most cases, we needed to re-examine the images ourselves to resolve the uncertainty. One could not determine from looking at the report whether the cancer was localized or had spread.

Consider the inefficiency of this approach: multiple research teams, each re-interpreting images in parallel with the existing conventional reporting process, just to capture information *that is essential to patient care and should already be in our reports.*

In the 1920s, Preston Hickey, an eminent radiologist from Detroit, had a similar crisis of confidence in the radiology report. Dr. Hickey had conducted an informal survey of radiology reporting for a surgical meeting by asking his colleagues from around the country to contribute samples of their reports. He expected his respondents to send their exemplary work. Unfortunately, he found that "in only a few cases were [the reports] worded [such] that the reader could form from the descriptions a diagnosis of the conditions present." He added: "If one wished to make a statistical study of the effect of different lines of surgical procedure in the treatment of fractures of the lower end of the radius, the handicap would be formidable."[5]

Sadly, almost 100 years later, little has changed. Clear and well-organized reports are useful not only for clinical care and research, but also for myriad other purposes, such as clinical performance improvement, resident education, and practice certification. Anyone who has attempted to glean definitive conclusions from even a small sample of radiology reports will agree we have a problem.

The Radiology Report at a Turning Point

"When I use a word," Humpty Dumpty said in rather a scornful tone, "it means just what I choose it to mean — neither more nor less."

"The question is," said Alice, "whether you can make words mean so many different things."
—*Lewis Carroll* [27]

The published literature is full of impassioned, often quixotic, editorials and letters to the editor arguing against a given word of dubious value, or inveighing against a particular phrase that lacks clarity. Although a few brief reporting guides are available, a major gap remains: there is no comprehensive source for the best thinking on how to create radiology reports.

I wrote this book to help radiologists produce better reports. This book collects the best thinking on how to report, conveying practical advice for precise image interpretation and clear communication. The reporting tips I provide will rely on evidence-based and time-honored truths, supported by relevant published literature when it is available. When formal or quantitative tools are available to help understand the report and its content, I will use them too. (But I promise: no complex equations and only a couple of Greek letters.)

But universal truths and evidence-based analysis have their limits. The radiology report tells a story and, like most narrative, ultimately is personal. Because rules for compelling storytelling are difficult to define, almost everyone has an opinion, often strongly held. As we sort through what constitutes a high-quality radiology report, I will alert you when the published evidence is thin. When evidential support is weak or controversial, I will highlight the best information from both sides so you can draw your own conclusions.

Airing these arguments and openly weighing the evidence will stimulate careful thought about your reporting habits. Through this dialogue, I expect we can forge a consensus on the important characteristics of an optimal radiology report, thereby enabling clearer communication and fostering a higher quality product for the referring clinicians and patients we serve. After all, that's what practicing medicine is all about.

A Guide for the Reader

This book is divided into three parts.

Part I, Practical Advice, is a how-to guide for inexperienced and veteran radiologists alike. It provides tips and insights on radiology report style and structure that will help any radiologist produce better reports.

Part II, History and Foundations, describes the historical, logical, and statistical underpinnings of radiology reporting. These chapters are aimed at readers with an interest in the theoretical and rhetorical foundations of the radiology report and the associated computational and decision-making formalisms.

Part III, The Future, predicts the role of the radiology report a decade from now, in a world with ubiquitous electronic medical records, pervasive collaboration tools, engaged patients, and new payment models.

Part I: Practical Advice

What is the best way to express an observation in an imaging report? Chapter 2, Expressing an Imaging Observation, focuses on the crux of radiology reporting: the imaging observation. Here, you will learn how to construct a sentence describing observations and their anatomic locations. Mastery of these techniques is the essence of radiology reporting.

Do you know when to use the word "normal"? Is "clinical correlation suggested" a frequent element of your reports? How do you express uncertainty? Chapter 3, Radiology Reporting Best Practices, reviews many common themes and problems in radiology reporting and provides evidence-based practical solutions that have stood the test of time.

Is "tumor" a synonym of "malignancy"? Is the thumb the first digit? What does it mean to call a structure "prominent"? Chapter 4, A Guide to Reporting Style, addresses stylistic and grammatical issues that arise frequently in the radiology report. These issues often are a matter of opinion. We will consider opposing views and suggest common-sense solutions.

Have your reports ever contained the phrase "bilateral bleak views" or "metacarpal fail and kill joints"? Chapter 5, Mastering Speech Recognition, reviews current speech recognition technology and provides tips to hone its performance. A functional understanding of these systems will yield methods for optimizing how they work for you on a daily basis.

Do you need help organizing the material in your reports? Chapter 6, Organizing the Radiology Report, outlines a standard master template for the structure and contents of a radiology report, listing widely accepted section headings and describing how report information should be divided among them.

Part II: History and Foundations

Why are radiology reports still in narrative form, while much of the medical record contains discrete concepts, like problems, medications, and allergies? Why has the radiology report remained a narrative while information technology has revolutionized many other industries? Chapter 7, The History of Radiology Reporting, provides context for current reporting tools by recounting the origins of many common reporting methods, including transcription, speech recognition, point-and-click reporting, and multimedia reporting.

Are you interested in standardizing your reports but don't know where to start? Chapter 8, Toward Structured Reporting, reviews the recent history and practice of structured reporting, and helps radiologists respond to the economic forces changing how radiology services are valued. This chapter contains practical advice for radiologists wishing to standardize their reports.

Do you need a guide for proper terminology in radiology reports? Chapter 9, Standard Terminology for the Radiology Report, describes the critical role that a standard vocabulary plays in a high-quality radiology report, using

BI-RADS® (Breast Imaging Reporting and Data System) as a model for the rest of radiology.

Are your reports as persuasive as they should be? Chapter 10, How to Think about Imaging Information, builds a logical foundation for the reasoning and rhetoric inherent in radiology reports. These principles provide vital tools to solve many reporting conundrums, and will be of special interest to those curious about the origins of probabilistic thinking.

We are all susceptible to cognitive errors that lead to flawed decision making. Chapter 11, Decision Making for Diagnostic Imaging, reviews optimal techniques for clinical decision making and highlights the mental mistakes that can afflict all human decision makers, including radiologists.

Part III: The Future

In 10 years, the radiology report will look strikingly different than it does today. Chapter 12, The Future of Radiology Reporting, contemplates future directions for radiology reports, from multimedia reporting to computer processing of natural language to machine learning and the future of radiology communication, including the possible extinction of the radiology report.

Special Features

Throughout the book you will find occasional practical tips, highlighted in gray. These tips point to information of immediate value in your practice, help resolve key controversies, and highlight the optimal role of information technology in radiology reporting.

Some of the material covered here is changing rapidly, such as the role of information technology in radiology reporting. To stay current, please refer to the companion web site for this book, http://radiologyreportbook.com, where updated information and supplementary material are available.

If you have comments or feedback on any aspect of this book, please send email to radiologyreportbook@gmail.com. Happy reading.

Part I:
Practical Advice

Chapter 2:
Expressing an Imaging Observation

There is no more difficult art to acquire than the art of observation, and for some … it is quite as difficult to record an observation in brief and plain language.
—*William Osler*[28]

Most radiology reports are composed of sentences. Someday, that may change. Until then, radiologists must answer two key questions: How should report sentences be organized? What information should they contain?

Short Declarative Sentences

To be simple is to be great.
—*Ralph Waldo Emerson*

I once worked with a master teacher who commonly dictated a normal radiographic study of the foot, in its entirety, as follows: "I see nothing abnormal in the foot." He emphasized a personal touch and an active verb. Starting with our first writing experiences in English class, we are drilled on the appeal of the active voice. But in most cases, the active voice of the radiologist needlessly personalizes clinical documentation and thereby undermines its authority. So forget what you learned in English class, and dictate instead, "The foot is normal."

The clearest reports are composed of short declarative sentences. Short sentences convey confidence. Clinicians prefer short sentences.[29] A consistent (and admittedly monotonous) set of present-tense verbs like "is" and connector words such as "is present in" are indispensable tools of this approach.

In this chapter, we will analyze the most common type of sentence that appears in the radiology report, which I will call an *observation sentence.* (Later, we will discuss other sentence forms, such as those that attempt to interrelate previously described findings or that enumerate a differential diagnosis.) Consider the following observation sentences taken from radiology reports:

> `"A cyst is present in the right ovary."`

> `"The heart is mildly enlarged."`

> `"A small left pleural effusion likely is present."`

> `"A focus of low attenuation is present in the temporal lobe."`

> `"On the post-contrast images, a 1-cm exophytic, enhancing mass likely is present in the anterior upper pole of the left kidney."`

These sentences have common elements, inherent in the nature of the radiology interpretation process.[30] Let's dissect the last example above. The essential element of an observation sentence is the observation itself, in this case, a "mass." The anatomic location of the finding is critically important, in this example, "the left kidney." Precision is added by modifying and refining the observation (e.g., "exophytic, enhancing") and its location (e.g., "anterior upper pole").

Most often, an observation "is present in" an anatomic location, as in the preceding example, but more complex spatial relationships between anatomy and pathology can occur, such as a mass "abuts" or "projects from" an anatomic structure.

Certainty is uncommon in radiology, so expressions of the likelihood that the observation is truly present are often required: In this case, that uncertainty is expressed by the word "likely." Finally, to assist others in locating key observations, it may be helpful to note where the observation can be found on the images, in this case "on the post-contrast images."

Figure 3 shows these key elements of an observation sentence. In the sections that follow, we will discuss each element in more detail.

Report Element	Example
Observation	Mass
Anatomic location	Left kidney
Relation	Arises from
Observation modifiers	1 cm
Anatomic modifiers	Anterior
Uncertainty	Likely
Location on the image	On the post-contrast images

Figure 3. Elements of a sentence that expresses imaging observations.

Tip: Most sentences in the radiology report describe what the radiologist observes on the images and use a small number of consistent elements.

A Spectrum of Imaging Observations

Examples: cyst, mass, pleural effusion, cardiomegaly.

It is ironic that radiologists have not consistently agreed on the word to describe the things we see on an image. Should we call them observations? Findings? Abnormalities? Images often depict devices, artifacts, and signs of aging that are not abnormal, so the term *abnormalities* is inaccurate. The term *finding* is too broad, because it signifies something that could have been "found" by a physical examination or a laboratory test, rather than through imaging. So in this book, we will use the term *observation* to represent the things we see on an image.

It is useful to consider imaging observations on a spectrum, ranging from nonspecific visual features, through identifiable pathophysiologic processes, to diagnostic disease classifications.[31] Visual features, sometimes called imaging signs, are the most basic imaging observations we can make and represent the shapes and shadows that hit our retina, such as "blunted," "plate-like," "smooth," or "spiculated." Identifying these basic visual features of the image doesn't require medical training—even a small child knows what they look like. Especially evocative visual features sometimes have been named for their discoverer, such as Rigler sign,[32] when air is present on both sides of the intestinal wall, or Kerley lines caused by fluid or cellular infiltration of the pulmonary interstitium.[33] But visual features rarely allow us to draw specific clinical conclusions.

Further along the spectrum of observations are pathophysiologic processes, whose presence may be suggested by one or more visual features. For example, a blunted costophrenic angle is often a sign of a pleural effusion, a pathophysiologic process. Platelike opacity in the lung usually represents atelectasis, another pathophysiologic process. And, an intestinal air-fluid level on an abdominal radiograph can be a sign of adynamic ileus. These pathophysiologic processes are often the signs of specific diseases and therefore represent the building blocks of differential diagnosis. Understanding how these processes create specific visual features requires not just medical education but radiology training.

At the most specific end of the observation spectrum are distinct diseases or diagnoses, such as pneumonia, gout, or adenocarcinoma. These diseases are defined by specific criteria, often based on tissue examination or an agreed constellation of clinical findings. When a specific group of visual features and pathophysiologic processes are seen together, we sometimes can conclude a disease is present. Radiologists should strive to make these disease-specific observations whenever possible because they often have clear implications for subsequent patient care.

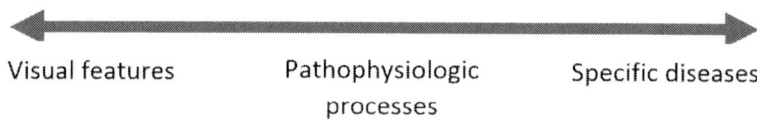

Visual features   Pathophysiologic   Specific diseases
                                processes

Figure 4. A spectrum of imaging observations representing a
range of clinical specificity.

Tip: Imaging observations can be viewed on a spectrum from visual features, through pathophysiologic processes, to diseases and diagnoses. Radiologists should strive to identify the presence of a specific disease if the observations allow.

Anatomic Location

Examples: right ovary, left kidney, left pleural space, heart, liver

The value of an imaging observation is enhanced by a precise anatomic location. We all learn human anatomy in medical school, so specifying anatomy in radiology reports is not a mystery. However, there are a few subtleties: Anatomic information can be contained in terms that combine both anatomy and pathophysiology, such as "cardiomegaly" and "hydroureter." And sometimes anatomic location is implicit in a pathologic observation, such as "ascites," "pneumonia," or "Budd-Chiari." But this attempt at brevity can be taken to extremes. An "effusion" observed on a chest radiograph could refer either to the pleural or the pericardial space. When in doubt, avoid such anatomic ambiguity.

Spatial Relationships

Examples: is present in, abuts, arises from, obstructs

Grammatically speaking, observations and anatomic locations are most commonly expressed as nouns, such as "mass" and "liver." How do these two critically important nouns relate to one another? To form a complete sentence, a verb is needed. A basic method to express the spatial relationship between an observation and its location is to use the phrase "is present in." For example, we report that "a mass is present in the liver." This simple locution is preferable to anthropomorphic verbs, such as "The liver *shows* normal size and contour" or "osseous structures *reveal* degenerative changes."[34]

Many other observations can be expressed by using a subject and an adjective with a linking verb. For example, when we report that "the spleen is enlarged," "spleen" is the subject and "enlarged" is the past participle, serving as an adjective that modifies the subject. When an imaging observation is expressed in this way, the present tense linking verb "is" can be used in most situations.

When necessary, more specific verbs or verb phrases, such as "abuts," "arise from," or "obstructs," can delineate more specific spatial relationships between anatomy and observation.

Tip: A narrative report sentence should contain anatomy and an observation connected by a simple verb phrase, typically "is present in" or "is." This parsimonious method of expression is equivalent to reporting methods that omit the verb, such as "Left kidney: simple cyst" or "Heart: mildly enlarged."

Observation and Location Modifiers

Examples: anterior, superior, mild, acute, 1 centimeter

Precise descriptions of both the imaging observations and the anatomic region are essential for an optimal imaging report. For example, rather than specifying just the left kidney, we can describe the *anterior superior* aspect of the *left upper pole*, to pinpoint the observations within a specific portion of the kidney.

Likewise, we can refine our observations with descriptions of their severity, acuity, or size. For example, we often describe *mild* congestive heart failure, an *acute* fracture, or a *1-cm* mass.

In most cases, these modifiers will serve as adjectives modifying the noun that specifies the anatomic location or the observation. However, for ease of reading, these modifiers can also be expressed in separate sentences. For example, "A 3-cm mass is present in the left upper renal pole. The mass is calcified."

Tip: Modifiers help us express refined descriptions of an observation and its anatomic location in one or more short declarative sentences.

Expressing Uncertainty

Examples: definitely is present, likely is present, may be present

Uncertainty is ubiquitous in diagnostic radiology. Even when the mass on the mammogram is obvious, the best radiologist may not be able to distinguish between a fibroadenoma and an invasive ductal carcinoma. Such uncertainty is inherent in the practice of medicine. Embrace it. The most successful imaging reports express uncertainty clearly and unambiguously, explicitly acknowledging that some conclusions cannot be made solely on the basis of the images.

Expressions of uncertainty in imaging reports most commonly refer to the presence or absence of the observation: "A mass may be present." But there are many other dimensions of uncertainty. For example, uncertainty may exist about the anatomic location: "The retroperitoneal mass may arise from the right kidney or the right adrenal gland." Or there may be uncertainty about the applicability of a modifier: "The mass may be calcified." Sometimes there is uncertainty about the spatial relationship between the observation and the anatomic location: "The mass likely extends into the inferior vena cava." In each of these cases, a radiologist shows strength by avoiding vagueness and hedging and by addressing the uncertainty explicitly and systematically with standard terms.

In Chapter 3, we will explore additional subtleties of expressing uncertainty, including the use of consistent phrases, such as "definitely is present," "likely is present," and "may be present."

Locating Observations on the Images

Examples: on the post-contrast images, on the lateral view, on the coronal T1-weighted pre-contrast images, on image 12 of series 4

In most cases, there is no specific clinical need to specify where on the images an observation is visualized. Nevertheless, such a courtesy is helpful to less experienced viewers who later need to find the imaging evidence for an assertion in the report. And sometimes, the location of an observation on an image can have diagnostic significance. For example, a nodular opacity seen only on a single radiographic view may represent a vessel on end rather than a pulmonary nodule. Likewise, visualizing an observation on a particular MR imaging sequence or on the post-contrast CT images can affect the differential diagnosis. In such cases, identifying the imaging location provides vital support for the diagnostic conclusions of the report.

Building a Rhetorical Foundation

To communicate, put your thoughts in order; give them a purpose; use them to persuade, to instruct, to discover...."
—*William Safire*[35]

We now turn our focus to the order in which observation sentences appear in the report. Sentence order is crucial to creating a coherent argument that supports the report's conclusions. Consider the following excerpt from a chest radiograph report:

> "There is blunting of the right costophrenic angle due to a small effusion. Mild diffuse pulmonary edema is present. The heart is mildly enlarged. These findings represent mild congestive heart failure. There is a platelike air space opacity at the right base, which is likely atelectasis caused by the effusion."

It is helpful to think of each sentence as one observation in a network of observations that support the conclusions of the report.[36] For example, the first sentence establishes the presence of blunting. The second sentence indicates that pulmonary edema is present. To illustrate the resulting relationships, each of the observations in this report has been placed in the semantic network shown in Figure 5. The dotted-line boxes indicate where each observation falls on the spectrum of observations we discussed earlier.

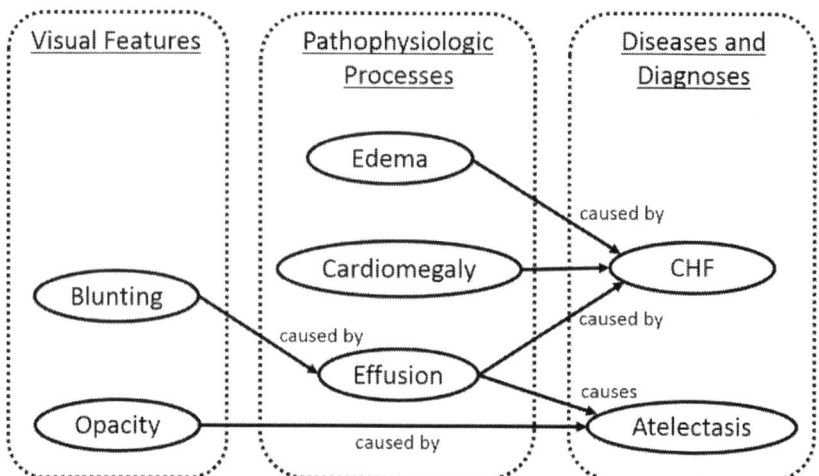

Figure 5. The semantic network of observations that corresponds to the above narrative report. *CHF* = congestive heart failure.

Establishing a similar thought process to organize your observations will help you create clear and persuasive reports. Begin by creating short declarative sentences for each observation. Then organize your observations to create a clear inference path from visual features to diseases.

Chapter 3:
Radiology Reporting Best Practices

Speak properly, and in as few Words as you can, but always plainly; for the End of Speech is not Ostentation, but to be understood.
—William Penn[37]

As a young second year resident, I once overheard an eminent radiologist—the author of a textbook you probably know—describing an abdominal radiograph as "marred by motion artifact." For some reason, the word "marred" stuck with me. I had seldom heard the word, and certainly never as part of a radiology report. This radiologist's reports often approached the poetic—composed of words we would have aspired to write in an English seminar.

And yet, alliteration and adjectival variety, while pleasant to the ear, may generate more confusion than clarity. Is "marred" worse than "limited"? Is "degraded" different than "marred"? Do these near-synonyms indicate that the exam should be repeated? Is it possible to use these terms consistently to express different levels of image quality? For a reader seeking information about the quality of the images, a small and consistent set of terms is less melodic but more useful.

Like varied terminology, varied sentence structure is a conundrum for radiology reporting. A spectrum of syntax engages the reader of a novel. But readers of our reports are not interested in literary style. Readers seek relevant clinical information and appreciate qualities such as clarity, brevity, consistency, and specificity.[38] In the sections that follow, I hope to help you "unlearn" some of what you learned in English class so you can optimize your reporting style.

Tip: Many of the writing techniques we learned in English class are the enemy of efficient information transfer and grind the gears of clinical communication.

Develop a Reporting Routine

Some things we want to do are simply beyond our capacity.
—*Atul Gawande*[39]

The last time you flew on a commercial flight, did it relax you to know that the cockpit crew used a checklist to configure the aircraft for takeoff? Although each pre-flight step is simple, recalling a long sequence correctly every time is well beyond the capacity of most humans. As radiologists, we face similar complexity every day. Even a subspecialized radiologist whose practice focuses exclusively on abdominal CT might face in rapid succession an exam for appendicitis, an exam after a major traumatic event, and an exam to stage pancreatic cancer. Reliably evaluating images from such diverse patients sometimes exceeds our capacity.

The best way to combat this cognitive overload is to follow a template to guide our routine, just as pilots do. When I report observations from a bedside chest radiograph, a template prompts me to describe the lungs, then the heart and mediastinum, next the tubes and lines, and finally to comment on whether a pneumothorax is present. The template fosters consistent reporting habits and reduces clinical complexity. The consistent ordering of information also helps report readers find and absorb the information they need—no wonder clinicians prefer such reports.[24,40,41]

Some will argue that templates and checklists undermine the sound rhetorical foundation that radiologists must construct to support a report's conclusions. They contend that an immutable ordering of findings hinders ranking of observations according to their importance and inhibits complex semantic linkages. But just as a pilot disengages the autopilot when encountering unusual flying conditions, the radiologist can depart from a standard template whenever the complexity of a case suggests the need for stylistic flexibility.

Another common concern is the effect of templates on trainees. Radiology residency programs sometimes worry that standard report templates serve as a crutch for trainees, who slip into habitual fill-in-the-blanks mode rather than using clinical judgment to analyze a constellation of observations. There is some truth to this critique. But this argument against checklists is analogous to the assertion that we should not learn to use computer calculators because we might forget our multiplication tables. We should learn to multiply, but attaining that skill shouldn't dissuade us from using a computer to solve critical or complex problems, because calculators reduce errors and improve accuracy. I am thankful that architects use computers to design our bridges.

Learning to analyze a case while being prompted by a template is an important skill in its own right. Over time, these routines become second nature and improve the performance of imaging professionals at all levels of expertise. Someday, a scholarly radiologist will address the important question of how report templates affect radiology education.

Tip: Develop a consistent reporting routine for each exam type on which you report.

The Virtues of "Normal"

> To study the abnormal is the best way of understanding the normal.
> —William James

The primary purpose of diagnostic imaging is to detect disease. As a result, radiologists occasionally view normal imaging studies as potentially inappropriate and a waste of time. But one of radiologists' most powerful contributions to patient care arises from their ability to rule out disease noninvasively. Many imaging exams are performed in the setting of low disease prevalence because there is a need to rule out serious problems, stop the work-up, and allay the patient's concerns.

Consequently, "normal" is one of the most powerful words a radiologist can use. "Normal" makes a sweeping statement by indicating, in singular fashion, that all abnormalities have been considered and excluded. Using "normal" will enhance your reputation among referring clinicians, because it gives them the two things they want most: a definitive answer that halts the work-up and good news for their patient. Frequent use of "normal" also provides a counterpoint to the reputation of radiologists as wafflers who hedge against the risk of an incorrect conclusion.

(Note: In the past, some have argued that under the right circumstances, the word "normal" should constitute the entire report.[30] But in today's world, a single-word report probably does not meet documentation requirements for most health care payers and is not acceptable to most referring clinicians.[42])

Tip: "Normal" is a powerful word. An exam interpreted as normal provides high value to the patient and reflects well on the radiologist.

"Normal" Impostors

Some will argue that no exam is truly normal, and that the word "normal" does not account for the panoply of variations among normal individuals. They argue that "unremarkable," "essentially normal," "relatively normal," "grossly normal" or some other variant would be more accurate. Let's discuss each of these impostors in turn.

When a trainee uses the term *unremarkable*, I highlight the inherent contradiction by asking: "If it's unremarkable, why are you remarking on it?" Perhaps I am being too literal. The American Heritage Dictionary defines unremarkable as "lacking distinction; ordinary." Is there a clinically meaningful distinction between those concepts and "normal"? I don't see it. Why not use "normal" instead?[43]

Imagine what goes through a reader's mind when a report states that the liver is "grossly normal" or "essentially normal." The referring clinician may think: In what nonessential ways does this patient's liver deviate from normal, and are they significant for the clinical decisions I must now make? Answering this question leads to a detailed reading of the body of the report, which leaves the question unresolved.

The use of "relatively normal" prompts the question: "Relative to what?" Relative to a younger patient? An older patient? Other patients who undergo this exam? This same patient's most recent exam? Again, the use of a qualifier sends the reader on a wild goose chase to delineate its meaning.

Some radiologists prefer to state that there are "no radiographically visible signs of disease." I suppose this locution is a hedge against abnormalities that are not detectable with imaging. From that perspective, stating "the heart is normal" in the report of a chest radiograph study is technically incorrect because radiographic images cannot demonstrate an arrhythmia, myocardial infarction, or valvular regurgitation—all significant cardiac abnormalities. I suppose this hedge could serve a purpose if the report reader knows nothing of the capabilities of radiography. But anyone who went to medical school must know that a chest radiograph will not show an arrhythmia, so the hedge has no real value.

"No significant abnormalities" and "normal for age" are two other frequent stand-ins for "normal." I suppose these apply when there are insignificant or age-related observations mentioned in the body of the report. But most people undergoing imaging are middle aged or older and have at least one benign abnormality, such as musculoskeletal degenerative changes, renal cysts, or vascular calcifications. Unless such observations are clinically relevant, I still favor "normal."

Tip: Avoid using substitutes for the term *normal*. Using "normal" whenever possible will enhance your reputation among referring clinicians.

Formal Disclaimers

Another manifestation of radiologists' fear of using the word "normal" leads to the inclusion of specific warning notices to referring clinicians in radiology reports. For example, a report might indicate that "occult scaphoid fractures may not be detected on routine wrist radiographs" or that "supine abdominal radiographs are not sensitive for the detection of free intraperitoneal air." In the era of automated speech recognition, these disclaimers can be incorporated into a standard template with minimal effort. Perhaps these statements have a role in educating referring clinicians—especially incorrigible ones—about the limits of our imaging procedures. But imagine that you were a referring clinician who often ordered these tests and had long ago internalized the lesson. The disclaimer would seem patronizing and would become repetitive over time. For this reason, other pedagogic strategies should be explored before these statements are employed. If they are employed, they should be used sparingly and reviewed frequently for their continuing value.

Within Normal Limits

A limit is defined as "a boundary surrounding a specific area." "Within normal limits" should be used only when adhering to that definition, not as a synonym for "normal." Describing a boundary only makes sense when observing a structure whose internal architecture cannot be discerned. For example, I use this phrase to describe the heart and mediastinum on a chest radiograph: "The heart and mediastinum are within normal limits."

Pertinent Negatives

I once overheard one end of a phone conversation between a curmudgeonly colleague and a referring clinician seeking the result of a head CT study. First, I heard the radiologist say "it was normal." Then, after a pause, he quipped, "Well, actually, there *was* a stroke, but I called it normal anyway." Apparently, the radiologist had failed to include the pertinent negative: "There is no evidence of stroke," prompting what he thought was an impertinent question warranting a sarcastic answer. This unfortunate and unprofessional encounter highlights a tension between referring clinicians and radiologists regarding the length and content of a normal report.

Pertinent negatives are findings we are looking for but aren't there. Rather than reading a one-word report, "normal," referring clinicians are reassured by reading: "The lungs are clear. The heart is normal in size. The mediastinal contours are normal."[44] This principle applies especially to more complex exams such as abdominal CT.[45] Pertinent negatives tell the referring clinician: "Yes, we looked." Pertinent negatives are particularly useful when they answer the referring clinician's query.[46] A specific response will enhance referring clinician satisfaction and create an ongoing incentive for the referring clinician to ask more specific clinical questions.

But excessive use of pertinent negatives has its drawbacks. Reports that contain long lists of pertinent negatives have a reassurance value but also take longer to read and process. For some screening exams, referring clinicians prefer a single-word report.[22] The tradeoffs between pertinent negatives and report length are best resolved through communication between report authors and report readers. If the readers know that any organ routinely visualized but not mentioned in the report can be assumed to be normal, they become much more comfortable with brief normal reports.

Tip: One exception to these principles of parsimony comes from a quirk of radiology billing. In some cases, a laundry list of normal organs must be included in the report for full payment. For example, in the United States, to be paid for a "complete" abdominal ultrasound study rather than a "limited" ultrasound study, several specific organs must be mentioned in the report.

Relevance: Making the Cut

No style of writing is so delightful as that which is all pith, which never omits a necessary word, nor uses an unnecessary one.
—*Thomas Jefferson*[47]

Your reader is in a hurry.[48] Every second, and every word, counts. Information relevancy should remain foremost in your mind as you choose what verbiage gets left out and what makes the cut. But relevance is a squishy notion, varying dramatically with context. How should you decide whether a finding should be highlighted by including it in the conclusions of the report?

Consider a patient with a mole on her left breast. To a dermatologist, that mole is his raison d'être. To a radiologist interpreting mammograms, that mole has no clinical significance other than its tendency to be confused with a breast mass. To ensure that the mole's shadow is identified and dismissed by others, it should be mentioned in the mammographic report. But should a cardiologist, who observes the same mole while listening to the patient's heart, mention it in the clinical note? Probably not.

The same spectrum of information relevance arises in the construction of imaging reports. Consider a patient with bulky spondylosis at the C7-T1 level. When observed on cervical spine radiographs obtained for radicular pain, the spondylosis may be causing the pain by compressing a nerve root and should certainly be highlighted. When that same spondylosis is seen on cervical spine radiographs obtained after a motor vehicle collision, it is a chronic finding that might explain the patient's pain but is unrelated to the trauma. It should be mentioned in the body of the report, but need not be mentioned in the conclusion. When cervical spondylosis appears on a lateral chest radiograph obtained for a chronic cough, many radiologists would not mention it at all, to avoid distracting readers from important cardiopulmonary observations.

In both of the examples above, the same observation may be the focal point of patient care, or it may simply be ignored, depending on the clinical context.[49] This dichotomy is another compelling reason for referring clinicians to provide a detailed clinical history when they order imaging studies.

Relevance issues also arise in the Summary section of the report. Some radiologists include all abnormal findings, no matter how insignificant, in the Summary. There is some merit to this approach, because there are times when the radiologist may have difficulty assessing the clinical significance of a finding. But this comprehensive approach tends to yield a long laundry list that dilutes the salience and impact of the most important information. A more selective approach avoids cluttering the Summary with information of limited utility to the referring clinician and emphasizes the truly significant findings. For example, in the Summary section of a chest radiograph study, the shoulder osteoarthritis need not be mentioned. Omit the simple cyst from the Summary of an abdominal CT study. And leave out the aortic calcification from the Summary of a lumbar spine radiograph study.

Tip: Prioritize the observations in your report. Irrelevant observations have a cost, paid by the distraction they cause from the salient information.

How to Say "I Don't Know"

When you know a thing, to hold that you know it; and when you do not know a thing, to allow that you do not know it; this is knowledge.
—Confucius[50]

Communicating uncertainty is the lifeblood of medical practice—especially for those who practice diagnostic imaging. One of my colleagues performed an ingenious experiment to illustrate the difficulties with expressions of uncertainty.[51] He conducted a computer search of radiology reports to find the 15 most common phrases that express diagnostic uncertainty. Then he asked radiologists and referring clinicians to rank the phrases according to the likelihood of disease they expressed, from least likely to most likely (Figure 6). Similar experiments have been performed in England[52] and on non-radiology narrative.[53]

The results show the vacuous nature of radiologists' common expressions: The same phrase can range in rank from nearly first to nearly last! And the opinions of referring clinicians were spread even wider.

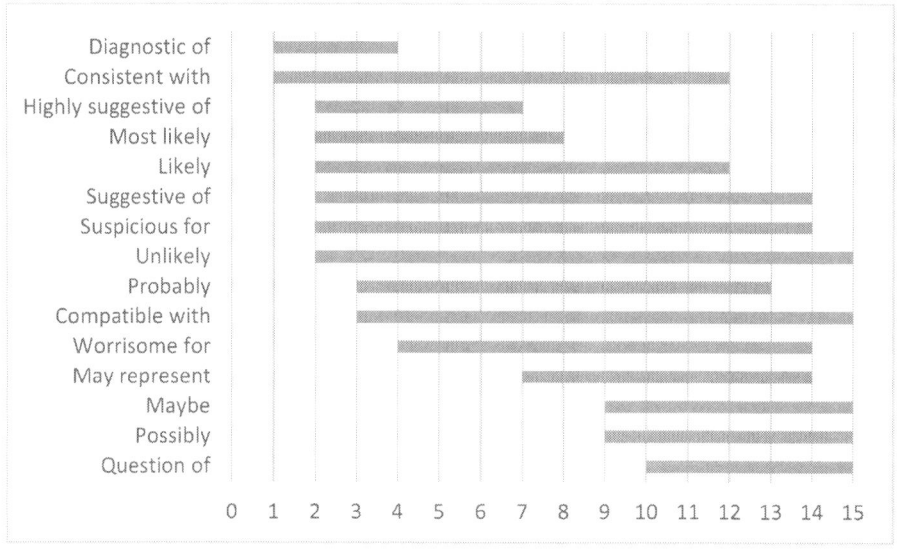

Figure 6. The ranges that radiologists ranked different expressions of uncertainty. 1 = most certain, 15 = least certain. The rank of one phrase ranged from first to twelfth. The ranges for non-radiologists were even wider. (Adapted from the Table in reference [51].)

Regarding physicians' ability to communicate uncertainty, you could say that the emperor has no clothes. Variety is the enemy of clarity. To promote consistency, I have adopted the systematic approach to the expression of uncertainty for reporting uncertainty shown in Figure 7.

Body of the Report	Summary
"A mass is present in the RLL…"	"RLL mass"
"A mass likely is present…"	"likely RLL mass"
"A mass may be present…"	"possible RLL mass"
"A mass likely is not present…"	"likely no RLL mass"
"No mass is present"	"no RLL mass"

Figure 7. Phrases corresponding to consistent expressions of uncertainty.

This scale is simple to learn because of its symmetry. And words such as "possible" and "likely" readily modify the verbs that appear frequently in radiology reports.

After using this scale for many years, I have learned to make occasional modifications. Sometimes, when I cannot say with certainty that an observation is present or absent, I nevertheless believe it is in the patient's best interest to halt the imaging work-up. I find the phrases "almost certainly present" and "almost certainly absent" serve this purpose well. The message is usually easily understood and well received by a wise referring clinician.

A similar problem occurs when a negative study is limited in some way (e.g., due to patient motion), but I nevertheless believe it is in the best interest of the patient to bring the work-up to a halt. "No definite evidence of a mass" preserves the symmetry of the scale and reduces the constraints inherent in just five distinct levels of likelihood.

The most unhelpful expression in the above scale is "likely is not present." A tentative denial of the condition that led to the exam in the first place always sounds limp and vacuous, and the referring clinician's uncertainty is bound to persist. The referring clinician often rightly thinks: "The report says probably not, but I'd better rule it out." To assist the referring clinician, I address the situation head-on by recommending the best next step in the work-up.[11]

Tip: Consistent expressions of uncertainty provide high-fidelity communication of the likelihood of disease, which referring clinicians will appreciate.

Uncertainty versus Vagueness

The true test of character is not how much we know how to do, but how we behave when we don't know what to do.
—John W. Holt, Jr.

Consider an experienced radiologist who observes a spiculated 1-cm nodule in the left upper lobe. The radiologist might assess the probability of cancer at 60%. The report might state:

```
This nodule likely represents lung cancer. A chest CT
with contrast is recommended for further evaluation.
```

On the other hand, a less well-trained radiologist, who is unable to assess accurately the chance of cancer or who is overly preoccupied with the risk of being incorrect, might intentionally obscure the likelihood with ambiguous terms and phraseology:

```
Diagnostic possibilities include cancer, non-calcified
granuloma, artifact, metastasis, or conceivably unusual
infection.  Because a tumor cannot be excluded, clini-
cal correlation is suggested and further work-up may be
of value.
```

Such vagueness is the malevolent counterpart of uncertainty, undermining clear communication and corroding the credibility of the radiologist. While some credit could be given for the list of differential possibilities, the report's verbosity and lack of actionable information constitutes a medicolegal risk and serves primarily to distract from the most likely and most important diagnostic possibilities.[54,55]

Reporting a Differential Diagnosis

In an ideal world, patients would be afflicted by only one disease at a time. But more commonly, multiple diseases may coexist and interact to explain the patient's malady and the associated imaging observations. Although use of a consistent uncertainty scale remains essential, reporting a differential diagnosis also requires deft phrasing. A few key principles can help to reduce the complexity of a long differential: Each possible diagnosis should be listed, using a consistent scale to express its likelihood.[56] The rationale for ranking one diagnosis above the other should be explicit, even when those reasons flow from the clinical history rather than the images themselves. For example:

```
These findings likely represent congestive heart fail-
ure.  Because there is no cardiac enlargement and the
patient is immune-suppressed, pneumocystis and other
atypical infections should be considered as less likely
diagnostic possibilities.
```

Formulating a rich differential diagnosis can be particularly challenging when inadequate clinical information is provided with the referring clinician's order. In those cases, I often use the phrase: "In the appropriate clinical setting, this could also represent…" to indicate that non-imaging factors strongly influence the likelihood of a diagnosis. Others rely on "clinical correlation suggested," which is a love-it-or-hate-it phrase that we will discuss later in this chapter. (Spoiler alert: I hate it.)

Tip: To report a differential diagnosis, supplement a consistent certainty scale with prose that makes the relative likelihood of each diagnosis transparent to the reader.

Uncertainty and Belief

Medicine is a science of uncertainty and an art of probability.
—*Sir William Osler*

If you ask a layperson what uncertainty means, he will usually describe something that we do not know for sure. An academic might define it more formally as a measure of belief that a conclusion is true. But when we discuss communicating about uncertainty, we need to consider two important alternative views of uncertainty: Are we communicating a measure of *change* in our belief that a disease is present (i.e., how strongly the imaging evidence supports the presence of disease) or are we communicating a post-test measure of belief (i.e., the likelihood that disease is present, given all the clinical evidence, including imaging)?

To illustrate the distinction between these two concepts, consider two diagnostic imaging examinations. The first is a mammogram. When a particular morphology of calcification leads a mammographer to assign a BI-RADS (Breast Imaging Reporting and Data System) Category 3, we know the precise chance of cancer in that lesion.[57] That crisp and accurate assessment of uncertainty is tantamount to specifying the post-test probability of cancer. When the relationships between imaging observations and disease likelihood arc well understood, as in breast imaging, the imaging report conveys the post-test probability of disease. (Note: In Chapter 10, we will discuss the formal definition of this quantity, the *predictive value* of the test.)

On the other hand, consider a radiographic study of the chest performed for suspected pneumonia. When an area of consolidation is present at one lung base, the features of the consolidation, including its morphology, margins, volume loss, and the presence of air bronchograms, can help to determine the likelihood that pneumonia is present. But clinical variables, such as the characteristics of the patient's sputum and the presence of fever or cough may supersede the imaging evidence. So expressing a post-test probability of pneumonia on the basis of the chest radiograph often is beyond the radiologist's capacity. In that situation, the imaging report should express the degree to which the images might *change* the belief that pneumonia is present. The referring clinician then can draw a more sweeping conclusion about pneumonia by combining the assessment in the radiology report with clinical factors that may be unknown to the radiologist. (In formal probabilistic terms, this corresponds to the *likelihood ratio* for the imaging information—also discussed in Chapter 10.)

Even better, both radiologist and referring clinician could spend some time discussing the evidence that each has about the case and coming to some consensus on the most likely diagnostic possibilities. When in doubt, pick up the phone.

Size Matters

It has been said that a radiologist with a ruler is a radiologist in trouble. Perhaps the trouble arises because appendages, organs, and intervals can vary greatly from person to person. Shaquille O'Neal wears a size 22 shoe. I wear size 10. Is there any reason to think that the width of our atlantodens intervals or the size of our spleens should be the same? Is there a single threshold above which these measurements, or any others, are abnormal for all individuals? Probably not. Part of radiology training is learning the varying appearances of normal and gauging the size of an anatomic structure relative to the size and proportions of the patient. The unthinking use of a ruler can sometimes become a substitute for good clinical judgment.

On the other hand, when the growth of an abnormality must be tracked closely over time, size should be expressed as a quantitative measurement. And plenty of reliable data are available on the range in which normal measurements typically fall.[58]

When a ruler is not needed, qualitative expressions of size, just like uncertainty and severity, should be expressed using a consistent scale. For my qualitative size scale, I use trace, small, moderate, large, and extremely large. Figure 8 provides examples of its use.

Size Phrase	Example
Trace	A trace right apical pneumothorax is present.
Small	A small left pleural effusion is present.
Moderate	A moderate amount of pelvic fluid is present.
Large	A large enthesophyte projects from the greater trochanter.
Extremely large	An extremely large lung mass invades the left inferior pulmonary vein.

Figure 8. Examples of a consistent qualitative size scale.

Extremely Small

I once reported a pneumothorax as "tiny" and was told by the referring clinician that the word was unprofessional. My first reaction was: Seriously?! But that comment has dissuaded me from using "tiny." Words with similar meaning include "minimal," "minute," and "diminutive." I use the word "trace" to signal that a pleural effusion, pneumothorax, or other abnormality is extremely small and probably not clinically significant. Until the radiology community can agree on one of these words, it is best to choose just one and to use it judiciously and consistently.

Too Small to Characterize

Cross-sectional images often demonstrate abnormalities that are too small to determine their pathologic origin. The phrase "too small to characterize" is useful in that situation, although the report should clarify what follow-up is needed for the lesion, if any. Please do not substitute the abbreviation "TSTC" or use this phrase as an adjective. For example, please avoid "There are three too-small-to-characterize lesions in the liver."

Enlargement Impersonators

When an anatomic structure is larger than normal, we say that it is "enlarged." This simple word, sometimes used with a measure of severity, such as "markedly enlarged," is all that is needed. Avoid stand-ins for "enlarged," such as "chunky," "plump," "generous," or the frequently used substitute, "prominent."

What does it mean to report that "the hila are prominent"? The American Heritage Dictionary defines "prominent" as "immediately noticeable; conspicuous." When we say that something is prominent, we are indicating it caught our eye. We are obligated to describe the reason for their conspicuousness. Are they larger than normal? Is their position or morphology abnormal? Do they appear brighter? If so, why?

Expressing Severity

All the grandest discoveries of science have been but the rewards of accurate measurement.
—*Sir William Thomson (Lord Kelvin)*[59]

Severity, like uncertainty, is one of the most common methods to qualify imaging observations. Although "mild," "moderate," and "severe" are almost universally used to express the extent of a clinical condition, they are not applied or interpreted consistently. To avoid this pitfall, I recommend that you associate specific severity levels with the constellation of findings seen in the condition in question. Figure 9 shows how particular imaging observations can be associated with the severity of cardiogenic edema on a chest radiograph.

Severity	Cardiogenic Edema Features
Mild	Vascular engorgement, interstitial edema
Moderate	Alveolar edema
Severe	Consolidation, bronchograms

Figure 9. A consistent severity scale for congestive heart failure.

Some radiologists prefer "marked" rather than "severe" because it avoids the ominous connotation of "severe." Others contend that "slight" should be used rather than "mild" when characterizing size (a particular form of severity).[60] Whatever words you choose, use them consistently. Convince your partners to use the same ones.

An even better approach is to adopt a grading scale from the published literature. For example, a well-validated scale is available for the grading of osteoarthritis.[61]

Grade of Osteoarthritis	Description	Reporting Term
0	No radiographic findings of osteoarthritis	None
1	Minute osteophytes of doubtful clinical significance	Minimal
2	Definite osteophytes with unimpaired joint space	Mild
3	Definite osteophytes with moderate joint space narrowing	Moderate
4	Definite osteophytes with severe joint space narrowing and subchondral sclerosis	Severe

Figure 10. A consistent severity scale for osteoarthritis.[61]

If no published scales are available, consider collaborating with your referring clinicians to agree on a severity scale that is mutually understood. (See reference [62] for an example.)

Tip: Use a consistent scale to express severity. If such a scale is not available, collaborate with referring clinicians to create one.

Locating the Summary

The end is in the beginning and lies far ahead.
—*Ralph Ellison*[63]

I was taught to put my conclusions at the beginning of the report (in a section we then called the "Impression"). This practice likely arose long ago, when most reports were dictated on "tank" systems that used a telephone connection to record a dictation for later transcription. (See Chapter 7.) These tank systems offered a phone number that referring clinicians could call to listen to the dictation before it had been transcribed. Listing the conclusions first put the headline up front and saved the listener time fast forwarding the recording.

Other radiologists are taught just the opposite: The intricacies of a cross-sectional exam can be difficult to hold in your mind all at once. How can the radiologist summarize the conclusions before the report has been created? Completing the body of the report first can serve as a prompt for the radiologist when summarizing the results. These factors are particularly true for complex studies.

As more reports are distributed electronically and the sections of the report are standardized, this distinction will fade. Flexible report display technologies will enable report readers to decide the order in which they prefer the display of report sections.

In the meantime, where should the meaty conclusions of the report be placed? Here is the case for placing the Summary first: Aside from the obvious advantage of placing the most significant information at the top, which many readers prefer,[20] composing the Summary first enforces discipline on the report author. Take-home points must be identified in advance. A complete interpretation and conclusion must be formulated before starting the body of the report, which promotes logical organization and a coherent narrative.[64] And even within modern systems, it saves time for the reader: When the Summary appears at the top, there is less need to scroll.

Tip: Agree with your colleagues on a consistent position for the Summary section of your reports.

Making Recommendations

Advice is like snow - the softer it falls, the longer it dwells upon, and the deeper it sinks into, the mind.
—*Samuel Taylor Coleridge*

A recent study showed that radiologists recommend follow-up in 12% of reports.[65] Referring clinicians, especially primary care practitioners, prefer receiving radiologists' recommendations,[66] as long as the recommendations are made with appropriate strength to avoid painting the practitioner into a corner—leading to follow-up that might otherwise be unnecessary. Sometimes, we can strongly recommend follow-up solely on the basis of the imaging observations and common sense, such as recommending a chest CT follow-up for an aggressive lung mass seen on a chest radiograph. At other times, we must acknowledge the limits of what we know. To recommend MR imaging of rotator cuff disease seen on a chest radiograph, we need to know the patient's lifestyle and physical limitations, the degree of discomfort, and many other factors unrelated to the radiographic appearance. Such a situation warrants a much weaker recommendation, if any is provided.

Figure 11 shows the spectrum of phrases I typically use to make recommendations.

Recommendation Phrase	Example Sentence
...is recommended...	A chest CT *is recommended* to determine whether this nodule represents lung cancer.
...should be considered...	If there is clinical suspicion of a pericardial effusion, an echocardiogram *should be considered*.
...may be an appropriate next step...	A pelvic MR imaging exam *may be an appropriate next step* in the imaging work up of this unexplained pain.
...may be helpful...	If there is continuing clinical concern, a repeat obstruction series *may be helpful* to distinguish these two possibilities.

Figure 11. A list of recommendation phrases and examples of their use. The first row in the table expresses the strongest recommendation; the last phrase expresses the weakest.

When radiologists have all the information needed to determine the next step, they should make definitive recommendations that can be ignored only in exceptional cases. For example, "A chest CT *is recommended* to determine whether this nodule represents lung cancer."

A less definitive recommendation can be used to raise a differential possibility that the referring clinician may not have considered, but that also cannot be diagnosed from the imaging exam. For example, a globular heart on a chest radiograph can be a sign of a pericardial effusion but is a nonspecific imaging sign. In that case, the report could state that "If there is clinical suspicion of a pericardial effusion, an echocardiogram *should be considered*." Although conditional, the recommendation can be specific about the conditions under which further imaging should be considered, rather than using the vague phrase, "if clinically indicated."[49]

Recommendations can serve an informational purpose when referring clinicians may have limited knowledge of the imaging work-up. For example, "A pelvic MR imaging exam *may be an appropriate next step* in the imaging work-up of this unexplained pain."

A less forceful phraseology can be useful when the next step is clear, but only if specific clinical factors are present. For example, "In the setting of posterior knee pain, MR imaging of the knee *may be helpful* to further characterize this abnormality." Or, "If there is continuing clinical concern, a repeat obstruction series *may be helpful* to distinguish these two possibilities."

These recommendations assist a referring clinician who might need help determining next steps but do not bind the referring clinician when the radiologist has insufficient clinical detail.

Tip: Referring clinicians will thank you if you use a recommendation of the appropriate strength, because you provide useful information without compelling them to obtain follow-up testing.

Suggesting Clinical Correlation

Wise men don't need advice. Fools won't take it.
—Benjamin Franklin

How would you feel if a requisition crossed your desk stating "Recommend examining the images carefully"? Many radiologists would find this insulting, since we are trained to carefully examine the images. It's what we do; our colleagues expect it. Likewise, referring clinicians are trained to order imaging tests and to correlate the results of those tests with other available clinical information. For that reason, "suggest clinical correlation" is often just as offensive to referring clinicians.[12,13,67] I avoid using this phrase whenever possible.

Some radiologists use this phrase as a cudgel to force the ordering practitioner to supply better clinical information. Others use it as a hedge to deflect responsibility back to the referring clinician. In that setting, it is commonly preceded by a long, unranked differential diagnosis. No wonder referring clinicians think the phrase is overused!

The key to avoiding the "clinical correlation" trap is putting yourself in the place of the referring clinician. First, be sure the condition under consideration can be correlated to clinical findings. If so, rather than making the vague recommendation to correlate clinically, you can provide a specific conditional statement to help the referring clinician draw the correct conclusion. For example: "If the patient has tenderness in this area, this osseous fragment likely represents a small avulsion fracture. Otherwise, it is likely due to old trauma."

In some situations, clinical correlation is useless and should never be recommended. The histologic origin of a cystic pancreatic mass cannot be determined from the characteristics of the patient's abdominal pain. If you are truly stymied by a lack of necessary clinical information, consider picking up the phone and having a conversation with the referring clinician.

Tip: The indiscriminate use of "clinical correlation suggested" is an annoyance to referring clinicians.

The "Cannot Rule Out" Hedge

Referring clinicians have a distinct dislike of reports containing the phrases "cannot rule out" or "cannot be excluded" because they often represent an unnecessary and annoying hedge. These phrases typically should be avoided,[68] but occasionally can play a role in communicating uncertainty: Sometimes an observation likely represents something benign, but the radiologist want to signal to the reader that a more serious condition may be present. When a patient with a history strongly suggestive of pneumonia (e.g., fever, purulent sputum, crackles at the right base) has what appears to be classic atelectasis at the right base, I report that it probably represents atelectasis and describe why. But in that setting, I think it is important to state that "This probably represents atelectasis, but pneumonia cannot be excluded." Depending on the clinical setting, it may be entirely reasonable to treat that patient for pneumonia.

Sentence Fragments

Most radiology reports are narratives composed of complete sentences: "The lungs are clear. A small left pleural effusion is present." Others contain a collection of non-sentences: "Lungs clear. Left pleural effusion." There often is a generational divide in this preference. I prefer complete sentences because they signal to the reader the degree of professionalism that was used in reviewing the images.

A mixture of sentence fragments and full sentences, such as "The lungs are clear. Left pleural effusion," is unacceptable. If non-sentences are used, I think it is best to format the report by body part:

```
Lungs: clear
Pleura: left effusion
```

The optimal format should be selected after close consultation with referring clinicians.

Associated Studies

Many reporting systems provide the opportunity for radiologists to dictate one report for multiple studies. For example, one report could describe studies of both the foot and the ankle in a trauma patient. When the body parts are related, associating two studies in a single report is good practice. Why describe a 5th metatarsal fracture twice, once in the report of the foot radiographs and once in the report of the ankle radiographs? Instead, associate studies of related body parts.

Summary of Reporting Best Practices

Below is a brief summary of the good reporting practices we have reviewed in the previous two chapters:

1. Develop a consistent reporting routine for each study type.
2. Document observations with short declarative sentences.
3. Refine anatomic locations and observations with modifiers.
4. Specify spatial relationships with a small set of phrases, such as "is present in."
5. Express size using consistent terms, such as "enlarged."
6. Employ severity ratings based on the presence of specific imaging observations.
7. Strive to show how visual features lead to pathophysiologic processes and diagnoses.
8. Report uncertainty with consistent terms.
9. Include a small number of pertinent negatives in your report.
10. Answer any specific clinical questions posed in the request.
11. Prioritize relevant observations. Less relevant observations detract from the important information.
12. Recommend follow-up with a strength appropriate to the situation.
13. Avoid using "clinical correlation suggested."
14. Embrace the word "normal."

Chapter 4:
A Guide to Reporting Style

Choose and arrange your words for the maximum effect on the reader.
—*The Random House Handbook*[69]

Mark Twain once penned a scathing essay on the literary offenses of James Fenimore Cooper.[70] Here are a few of his critiques:

1. Say what he is proposing to say, not merely come near it.
2. Use the right word, not its second cousin.
3. Eschew surplusage [excess].
4. Not omit necessary details.
5. Avoid slovenliness of form.
6. Use good grammar.
7. Employ a simple, straightforward style.

Much of Twain's pithy advice applies not only to 19th century novels, but also to 21st century radiology reports. But you needn't sound like Hemingway or Faulkner to be an outstanding radiology report author. Radiology reporting follows different rules than those you learned in English class, and stylistic choices are often subjective. This is the realm of personal opinion.

What follows are my views, in no particular order, on radiology reporting hot topics. I hope the following sections will stimulate thought and discussion and help you become a better radiologist and communicator.

Choose Your Words Carefully

Prefer the specific to the general, the definite to the vague, the concrete to the abstract.
— William Strunk and E.B. White, The Elements of Style[71]

The Images about Which We Report

When a patient lies on the CT table and images are obtained, what do we call the result? A CT study? A CT examination? A CT procedure? These terms are near synonyms. But to the uninitiated, frequent switching among them can cause confusion. "Examination" or "exam" connotes something similar to what happens to an ear with an otoscope. "Procedure" works well for interventional studies but sounds a little grandiose for the humble chest radiograph. In this book, we use "study," which is the generic term used by the widely adopted DICOM (Digital Imaging and Communications in Medicine) standard to indicate the set of images that result from a referring clinician's request.

Can You See an X-Ray?

The term *x-ray* is overused in hospitals today. "The patient is in x-ray." "Did you find the x-ray?" "I'm going to take your x-ray." None of these senses of the word correspond to the most accurate definition of "x-ray": a photon of a certain wavelength and frequency.[72] To avoid all this confusion, I prefer the term *radiograph* to indicate the images created by projecting x-rays through the patient. This term is becoming more widely accepted as we move into the digital era, and "film" is no longer accurate. Some prefer "conventional radiograph," or "ordinary radiograph,"[73] but there is nothing conventional or ordinary about it, so I prefer simply "radiograph." Combined with the reasoning in the previous section, I call it a "radiographic study" of a particular body part.

Confusion about Density

In the past, it was common to hear the term *density* to describe a bright spot on a filmed planar image. Density relates to the quantity of something per unit of space. Presumably, the word "density" refers to the properties of the tissue being imaged, rather than the image itself. But a planar radiographic image is a negative image (i.e., the image is brighter in areas where fewer photons hit the detector). The density of silver grains on a film is actually lower in brighter areas.

To clear up this confusion, some have used the term *radiodensity* to indicate that the tissue of interest is more "dense" to radiographic photons. Others have advocated the use of "shadows," which clearly connotes something that obstructs a beam of energy, in this case, x-rays. Another similar locution is to describe "markings" on the film, such as the "vascular markings" on a chest radiograph,[74] although there is some controversy over the utility of this term.[75]

I prefer the terms *opacity* or *radiopacity* (and their opposites, *lucency* and *radiolucency*). An "opacity" is something that is opaque or impenetrable by light or another form of radiant energy.[76] So "opacity" and "radiopacity" clearly convey that the tissue being imaged is opaque to x-ray photons, thereby causing a bright spot on the radiographic image.

Film versus Image

I have spent the last decade trying to eradicate the word "film" from my dictation vocabulary—with only limited success. Many radiologists now are young enough to have never worked with film and have nothing to unlearn. The rest of us must remember that "film" is an archaic method for capturing and storing an image that involves the use of silver grains and a substrate. Most images are now viewed on a computer screen. So if you are referring to a single image, please use "image" or "view" rather than "film." The scientific radiology journals have likewise been modernizing their terminology.[77]

Archaic Terms

The chief virtue that language can have is clearness, and nothing detracts from it so much as the use of unfamiliar words.
—Hippocrates

Certain terms are passed down from senior radiologists to trainees, with the original meaning lost in translation.[14] Few radiologists say "flat plate" or "roentgenogram." "KUB" is also archaic. It originally stood for "kidneys, ureters, and bladder," but it is still occasionally used as a synonym for a frontal radiograph of the abdomen.

Decades ago, films were developed by hand, using vats of developing solution, followed by a lengthy drying time. If an urgent reading was required before the film was dry, it was literally a "wet reading." Today, that term makes little sense. It is better to call it an urgent reading or even a STAT read.

Escape the Muddled Middle

A witty colleague once declared that the radiology logo should depict a weasel eating a waffle under a hedge. Some radiologists go out of their way to avoid commitment, using vague weasel words, waffling between conflicting interpretations, or hedging their bets. Readers of our reports have reason to be upset. Here are some tips to avoid these pitfalls.

The Observational Detachment Hedge

Image interpretation involves visual perception, which in many ways is intensely personal. It is tempting to bring ourselves as observers into the reports we create. Phrases such as "...are seen," "...are identified," "...appears," and "note is made of..." frequently can be found in radiology reports. Unfortunately, the author of such a report seems to be hedging by hinting at his or her own limitations: "If there were a more perceptive radiologist nearby, he or she might be able to see an abnormality, but I can't."[43] This approach insidiously deflates our referring colleagues' confidence in our interpretations. I call any such phrase an "observational detachment hedge." These hedges should be avoided, with one small exception: when the images are of limited quality. In that setting, observational detachment perfectly conveys the perceptual limitations at play and signals that significant abnormalities may be missed.

Severity Straddling

"South-southwest" is a precise point on the compass midway between south and southwest. When you read "mild to moderate osteoarthritis" in a radiology report, do you think of that precise point midway between mild and moderate, or do you think of a broad range that includes most of mild and most of moderate?[34]

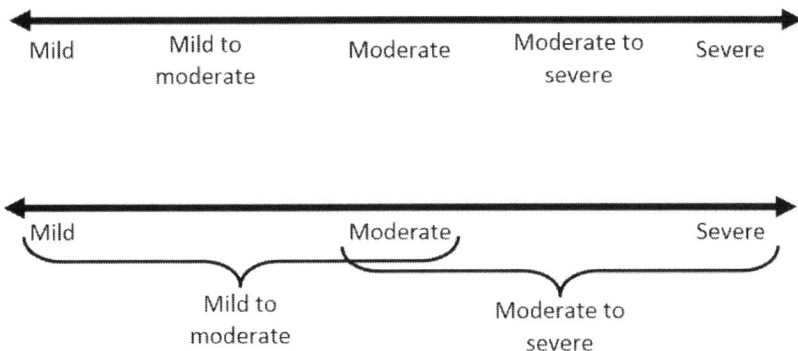

Figure 12. Top, what many radiologists intend when they dictate "mild to moderate" or "moderate to severe"; the interpolated severities represent the midpoint between two other expressions of severity. Bottom, what most radiologists are actually conveying by straddling severities—a broad and ill-defined range.

In my experience, the composite terms are less specific; few of us can reliably apply five levels of severity. I find it challenging to use just three levels of severity with consistency and recommend against hyphenating or interpolating.

Content-Free Sentences

The great art in writing well is to know when to stop.
—Josh Billings

Information seekers thrive on information density. An information-dense report is a highly efficient method of information transfer. Any excess verbiage in a report can obfuscate or dilute communication of the most important information. For the sake of the reader, avoid including sentences that convey no meaningful information to the reader and just take up space. For example:

```
There are no additional findings.

No other abnormalities are present.
```

Pause to reflect before dictating sentences like these.

Ambiguous Associations

A common form of imprecision in radiology reports is the mention of an association, without specifying the strength of the association or the direction of causality. For example, many reports state that one observation is "consistent with" or "in keeping with" another, as in "these erosions are consistent with gout" or "this deformity is in keeping with the patient's history of a fracture."

Observation A may be "consistent with" observation B, but we should make clear whether A causes B, B causes A, or a third factor, C, tends to increase the likelihood of both A and B. Statisticians and epidemiologists spend a great deal of time sorting out these causal patterns because they are essential to clinical reasoning and decision making. When possible, radiologists should do the same. For example, "these erosions likely are caused by gout" or "this deformity is due to a healed fracture." Your reports will be clearer when they include specific details about how two concepts interrelate.

The Self Referential Summary

> *Ma il mio mistero è chiuso in me (My secret is hidden within me)*
> —*Calaf, in Puccini's Nessun Dorma*

The purpose of the Summary or Impression section of the report is to highlight and summarize the most important observations, in order of priority. "Findings as described above" is *not* an appropriate summary.[43] If the report contains only disparate insignificant observations, none of which relates to the clinical question, consider using "no significant abnormalities," or even "normal."

Likewise, "No change" is an inadequate summary.[56] Many report readers are not following the case closely and will want to know: What has not changed? Refer back to the body of the report if you must, but please force yourself to include a brief conclusion.

Words to Avoid

Certain words, discussed below, should be used sparingly in the radiology report.[78–80]

Nonspecific

"Nonspecific" can be interpreted in many different ways. This phrase is especially popular among residents,[81] perhaps used as a crutch when they can't decide whether a study is abnormal. For example, "the bowel gas pattern is nonspecific." Some radiologists think nonspecific means the study is essentially normal. Others believe the term means the patient has either a mechanical obstruction or an adynamic ileus.[82] To make matters worse, referring clinicians have similarly disparate opinions, which vary from those of radiologists.[83]

Presumably "nonspecific" is intended to refer to the "specificity" of an observation in a statistical sense. (See Chapter 10 for a discussion of specificity.) In other words, "the bowel gas pattern that I see does not suggest any specific disease or pathophysiologic condition." But that raises a question: How is that definition different from normal? If the bowel gas pattern does not suggest that the bowel is normal, ask yourself why not and include the answer in your report. Otherwise, I suggest calling it "normal."

Borderline, Equivocal, and Top Normal

The use of "borderline cardiomegaly," "equivocal cardiomegaly," or their close cousin, "top normal" heart size, suggests the radiologist cannot decide whether cardiomegaly is present. These three terms are often used when the radiologist is on the fence between two conclusions and has doubt about the clinical consequences of the abnormality. Admittedly, the diagnostic criteria for cardiomegaly, and for many other conditions, can be vague and subjective. But that subjectivity also gives the radiologist the leeway to draw a conclusion without fear of being contradicted by a more definitive measurement of cardiac size. If the issue is a difficult imaging diagnosis that should be confirmed with a more definitive subsequent study, why not say it that way? Otherwise, get off the fence.

Suspicious and Indeterminate

The terms *suspicious* and *indeterminate* should be avoided if possible.[67] These words are similar to the "borderline" family described above, but they convey a higher likelihood of harm to the patient and a greater sense of urgency. "Suspicious" is a description of the viewer, not the image. If the likelihood of disease cannot be clearly quantified due to a lack of information or limited study (i.e., the presence of disease is "indeterminate"), some explanation should be given for the equivocation and what might be done to resolve the uncertainty. (Is this the wrong study? Is there an inherent limitation of this study? Is there a better alternative to imaging?) A clear likelihood scale (see Figure 7 in Chapter 3) is the preferred method to express uncertainty.

Irregular

What does it mean to say that a mass has an "irregular" border? Is the border ill-defined? Is it a mixture of lobulations and spiculations, partially obscured by other structures, or marked by angulation and changes in direction? Any of these more specific descriptions would be more helpful than simply calling it "irregular."

Emotional Content

> *May you live in interesting times.*
> —*Chinese curse (attributed)*

One truism we all learn in medical school is that it is a curse to be an interesting patient. In my opinion, "interesting" is only one of many temptations to sneak emotional content into a radiology report. While we certainly should empathize with our patients, emotional content in radiology reports tends to be distracting and can be detrimental to patient care. The radiology report should contain a precise expression of the facts, as best they can be determined from the data acquired.

What is the following sentence trying to convey?

```
No doubt, these findings indicate...
```

Perhaps it attempts to communicate the lack of doubt by the person interpreting the image. But why bring up doubt at all?

```
Surprisingly, there is no evidence of...
```

An expression of surprise may be highlighting the absence of an imaging manifestation that would be expected given the presence of disease, which makes this an atypical case. If that is the point, why not say it that way? Let's stick to the facts and leave our emotions behind.

Positive, Negative, and in Between

The Ambiguity of "Positive"

To say a CT study is "positive for liver metastases" has an awkward and paradoxical connotation. Remember that the patient, and those caring for the patient, may not share your view that the observation is a "positive" one. In fact, this phraseology may cause clinical confusion. For those reasons, I tend to avoid using "positive" and "negative" (except for special cases, such as to document ulnar variance). I prefer the alternatives, "present" and "absent."

Impertinent Negatives

> *Focusing is about saying "no."*
> —Steve Jobs

There are an infinite number of observations that are not present on an imaging study. So how should we decide which ones to mention? We typically use the notion of a pertinent negative: something that relates directly to the patient's clinical history or the reason for the exam, that we looked for but wasn't there. For example, "There is no evidence of pneumonia." Or, "There is no evidence of bowel obstruction or adynamic ileus." The search for these observations is often the main purpose of the exam because it answers the question being asked by the referring clinician.

A second vital purpose of negative imaging observations is to reassure the reader. You might occasionally get away with a one-word report of a preoperative chest radiograph study ("Normal"), but it is doubtful that same report would be tolerated for an abdominal CT study.[42] For a chest radiograph study, I say "The lungs are clear. The heart is normal in size. The mediastinal contours are normal." There is no harm in including this small number of sentences because they are designed to reassure: Yes, we looked. But as the number of negative sentences grows, beware that such clutter can distract from any significant positive observations. So keep the negatives brief, consistent, and clinically relevant.

Gratuitous Pessimism

> *You cannot climb the ladder of success dressed in the costume of failure.*
> —Zig Ziglar

Would you trust a report whose first sentence cites a failure? Worse than impertinent negatives are gratuitous negatives that encourage a depressing view of our capabilities: "The exam fails to reveal any evidence of pneumonia" suggests this study made an inferior contribution to the care of this patient. Yet a normal exam often enhances patient care by stopping the workup and is often just what the patient and referring clinician want to hear.[46] (See Chapter 3.) So let's keep it positive: (We are pleased and proud to report that) "No pneumonia is present."

Eschew Formality and Pomposity

The learned fool writes his nonsense in better language than the unlearned, but still 'tis nonsense.
—Benjamin Franklin

Latin Forms and Plurals

Because Latin forms are less well known than their English equivalents, they should be used only when there are no suitable alternatives. Here are situations where Latin is necessary: "data" is the plural of "datum"; "phenomena" (as in "vacuum disk phenomena are present in the lower lumbar spine") is the plural of "phenomenon," and "phalanges" is the plural of "phalanx." On the other hand, I prefer "femurs" to "femora," "granulomas" over "granulomata," the "deep femoral artery" rather than the "profunda femoris artery," and "vertebral bodies" instead of "vertebrae."

Abbreviations and Jargon

Abbreviations and jargon save space and can serve as useful shorthand when a complex term is used repeatedly. However, most complex terms are used only a few times in each report, negating this rationale. In the era of speech recognition, dictating "congestive heart failure" is not much more difficult than dictating "CHF" and is more likely to be recognized by the computer. Dictating "mets" for "metastases" also confers few communication benefits. Patients increasingly have electronic access to their reports and may be unfamiliar with abbreviations and jargon, so they generally should not be used in radiology reports.

Eponyms in Radiology

Fame is a series of misunderstandings surrounding a name.
—Joni Mitchell

Wouldn't it be grand to have a disease named after you? What a wonderful way to honor an important scientific discovery. Unfortunately, today's radiologists are probably too late to earn an eponym. The extinction of eponymous naming, at least in radiology reports, is probably a good thing, since our clinical and radiology colleagues, as well as our patients, appreciate simple descriptive names. For example, a Jones fracture is a short description, but your reader might not understand. Is the eponym really better than describing an oblique fracture through the metadiaphysis of the fifth metatarsal? Whenever possible, be descriptive.

There are some situations in which an eponym cannot be replaced, because the eponymous naming of diseases and syndromes was so common in the early 20th century. Some of those names, such as Crohn's disease, have a specific meaning for which synonyms are scarce. "Inflammatory bowel disease" is close to Crohn's disease, but this term is more general because it also includes ulcerative colitis. Since there is no single descriptive term for Crohn's disease, and the eponym is widely known, its use seems sensible.

The current trend is toward the omission of both the apostrophe and the "s" at the end of eponyms.[84] So hereafter in this book, we will do the same. Welcome to the world of "Crohn disease."

Repetitive Redundancy

It seems that perfection is attained not when there is nothing more to add, but when there is nothing more to remove.
—*Antoine de Saint Exupery*[85]

One of my favorite article titles is "A surfeit of superfluous and redundant pleonasms."[79] It targets numerous neologisms for elimination from the radiology report. In the examples below, the underlined portion can be omitted without altering the meaning. As we have emphasized elsewhere, information seekers prefer dense information, so avoid including words that don't add meaning.[15]

<u>Interval</u> change

Mass <u>lesion</u>

<u>Prior</u> history

Oval <u>in shape</u>

Small <u>in size</u>

<u>It was found that</u>

<u>It was demonstrated that</u>

<u>It is important to note that</u>

Perforate <u>through</u>

<u>Close</u> proximity

<u>Total</u> occlusion

The <u>bilateral</u> kidneys

<u>Aged</u> 56 years old

<u>Completely</u> asymptomatic

It's Ancient Greek to Me

> *Think like a wise man but communicate in the language of the people.*
> —*William Butler Yeats*

It is honorable to pay homage to the traditions of our teachers and elders. For this reason, many of us mimic certain aspects of their dictation style. By all means, imitate the experts, but try to omit the archaic and sometimes pompous constructions that are less familiar to the current generation of referring clinicians.

Dilation not "dilatation." — The American Heritage Dictionary gives essentially the same meaning for both of these words, although the latter is used only in medicine. So why not spare the two characters, the extra syllable, and the difficulties of being understood by lay people: Use "dilation."

Method not "methodology." — "Method" has been used in both common and scientific parlance for over a century, although "methodology" connotes the method for a formal scientific experiment and is more difficult for lay people to understand. Before using "methodology," check whether "method" is sufficient to capture your meaning.

Centimeter not "sauntimeter." — This one doesn't show up in the written report. But do we really need to pronounce the word centimeter as if we grew up in the British aristocracy?

Inventing New Words

> *A very great part of the mischiefs that vex the world arise from words.*
> —*Edmund Burke*[86]

Many imaging signs have taken on pithy designations, either through metaphor or through eponymous association.[87] Consider the following: football sign, apple core lesion, rugger jersey sign, tree-in-bud sign, signet ring sign, drooping lily sign. These metaphoric phrases are visually evocative. And every radiologist should be familiar with their appearance and their differential diagnosis. However, they are not taught to most non-radiologists and have limited communication benefit in the radiology report.

It is even more confusing to invent new words or phrases, since only you can know the definition of the neologism you have created.[34] For example, I challenge you to find a dictionary definition of "penciling" or "saucerization."[15] If you do find a source for the meaning of these terms, I suspect they will have very little to do with medical imaging and a great deal to do with sketch artists and pouring milk for stray cats. May I suggest "eroded to form a point" or "a concave erosion"? Invented visual analogies can be a useful pedagogic tool among radiologists. But for everyone else, it is preferable to use descriptive language.

Don't Call Me "-Al"

You may have noticed that the premier radiologic scientific and educational organization is known as the Radiological Society of North America (RSNA). Yet, the more common usage when describing something that pertains to radiology is "radiologic." The difference is one of history. The "-ic" suffix is sufficient to create the adjectival form of the word. The "-al" is redundant but was common decades ago, when the RSNA was formed. Unless the RSNA decides to change its name, it probably will continue to be known as the "Radiological" society. But for the rest of us, why not save a couple of letters and a redundant syllable, and drop the "-al"?[15] The same argument can be made for pathologic, obstetric, histologic, etc.

Specific Clinical Situations

Malignant Neoplasms

Don't use words as memorized formulas. Consider what they actually represent.
—Steven Pinker[88]

Word origins can be the key to clarity in medical discourse. Consider the following related words: *cancer*, *tumor*, *malignancy*, and *neoplasm*. We sometimes erroneously use these words as synonyms, but to avoid confusion, their subtle differences should be recognized.

Cancer is a word that is widely understood within both the medical and lay communities, for example, "lung cancer." Some use the word carcinoma as a synonym for cancer, but as we all know, carcinoma is a cancer of epithelial origin. There are many cancers that originate from other cell types, such as an astrocytoma. Cancer is an evocative term that clearly calls to mind this diagnosis. It can be supplemented by cell type if necessary.

Tumor is well understood by the lay public, but the term has the least specific clinical meaning. As many of us remember from medical school, the key signs of bacterial infection are tumor, dolor, and calor, Latin for swelling, pain, and warmth. Remember that a tumor need not always be a malignant neoplasm.

Malignancy is a noun derived from the commonly used adjective "malignant" and conveys aggressiveness and malicious intent. Yet, we sometimes

63

speak of malignant infections or other conditions. If you must use this word to describe cancer, use the more specific "malignant neoplasm," rather than "malignancy" alone.

Neoplasm comes from the Greek for "new formation." When using this locution, we must remember that not all neoplasms are malignant—or even cancer, for that matter. When a report intends to sound an alarm about a malignant neoplasm, it is helpful to use the word cancer or to pair the word with the cell type of origin to clarify its aggressiveness.

Finger Names

Hold up your hand and point to your first finger. Did you point to your index finger or your thumb? Probably some readers pointed to each. Finger numbering is ambiguous and can be confusing.[89]

All of these problems are best solved by referring to the digits by their standard names: thumb, index finger, middle/long finger, ring finger, and small finger. This naming method has been endorsed by the International Federation of Societies for Surgery of the Hand Research and is better understood than any other method.[90] Nobody will ask which finger is the index finger. If you must use numbers, pair them with the less ambiguous "digit" or "ray" rather than finger.

Fracture and Dislocation

Bones fracture; joints sublux or dislocate. So avoid describing hip fractures, shoulder fractures, or knee fractures. Also avoid "shoulder separation," which is a common locution for widening of the acromioclavicular joint due to ligamentous injury. These descriptions are insufficiently precise.

The Fine Points of Location and Laterality

Confusion can arise in the specification of medial and lateral when reading certain musculoskeletal studies. In the distal forearm, we might normally think of findings near the distal radius as being medial, but lateral is correct. Anatomic position is defined with the palms facing front, so the thumb is lateral, and the small finger is medial; the radius is lateral, and the ulna is medial. To avoid this confusion, use the unambiguous terms *radial* and *ulnar* in the upper extremity, rather than "medial" and "lateral."

The opposite advice applies when interpreting a study of the clavicle. Proximal and distal are sometimes interpreted relative to the shoulder joint but are also used relative to the central axis of the body. So medial and lateral are unambiguous and preferable ways to describe parts of the clavicle.

Getting Your Ducts in a Row

Similar confusion can arise when identifying precise locations within the biliary tree.[91] Many radiologists conventionally refer to the portion of the duct draining into the duodenum as the "distal duct," perhaps taking the perspective of pancreatic secretions. But through an endoscope, the ducts in the pancreatic tail are "distal" to the observer. To avoid ambiguity, it is best to locate the duct according to the portion of the pancreas it traverses, such as "the duct in the pancreatic head."

When referring to the position of one ductal observation relative to another, the terms *upstream* and *downstream* are unambiguous and should be used to describe relative position. Finally, remember that there is no anatomic structure called "the common duct." Be specific about whether you are referring to the common hepatic duct or the common bile duct.

A Bone to Pick

The word "ossific" derives from the Latin *os* for bone and *facere* for make. It implies an ossification *process*. This connotation is very appropriate for heterotopic ossification but not descriptive of a small opacity that may represent a fracture fragment.

Two better words are "bony" and "osseous," which are essentially synonyms of one another, signifying something composed of bone.[92] Because of its brevity and clarity, the plural noun "bones" is preferable to "osseous structures."[43] When an adjective is needed, bony is better understood by the lay public but carries a somewhat negative connotation, since the anatomy of some unattractively thin people is referred to as "bony," as in "get your bony ___ out of here." For that reason, I prefer "osseous," but I can't fault anyone for using "bony."

And please remember the distinction between calcific and osseous opacities. The latter has a cortex and trabecula; the former does not.

Bone Density

Radiologists who trained when I did in the early 1990s learned to make qualitative judgments about adult bone density on conventional radiographs. We use "osteopenia" to represent mild to moderate loss of bone density and "osteoporosis" to signify severe loss.[93]

As better tools to assess bone health have been developed, such as dual energy x-ray absorptiometry, quantitative CT, and ultrasound, we can now take a more rigorous approach to the assessment of bone density. These technologies can measure bone density as a percentile, called a T-score, which measures a patient's bones compared with those of a young normal reference population, or a Z-score, which measures bone density relative to age-matched controls.[94] This new ability to quantify bone density has led to quantitative standards for terminology, established by the World Health Organization.[95] (See Figure 13.)

World Health Organization (WHO) Criteria for Osteoporosis	
Term	T-Score
Normal	More than −1.0
Osteopenia	Between −1.0 and −2.5
Osteoporosis	Less than −2.5

Figure 13. World Health Organization criteria for osteoporosis. (Adapted from reference [95].)

This consensus terminology is based on a worldwide standard and should be adopted for all adults. The casual use of these same terms as we report conventional radiographs should be eradicated, because radiographs do not provide valid measures of bone density. For adults, "demineralization" and the more specific "diffuse bone loss" are preferable terms to describe low bone density on radiographs.[93] (This recommendation does not apply to pediatric radiographs, for which meaningful distinctions often can be made by examining the growth plates.[96])

The Meaning of "Infiltrate"

When I trained as a medical student on the West Coast many years ago, the word "infiltrate" was a synonym for "pneumonia." When I traveled to the East Coast for internship and residency, "infiltrate" meant something different: an air-space opacity that could represent either atelectasis or pneumonia (or presumably something else entirely). You can imagine the confusion that may result.[97]

According to the Fleischner Society[98]:

...「infiltrate」 remains controversial because it means different things to different people. The term is no longer recommended, and has been largely replaced by other descriptors. The term "opacity," with relevant qualifiers, is preferred.

I rest my case.

Distention and Dilation

In describing the bowel, please remember the distinction between distention and dilation. The colon is distended when it looks like it does during a barium enema study. The colon is dilated when its diameter is larger than that. Bowel dilation suggests intestinal obstruction; distention does not.

Die Contrast Dye

Dye is a substance used to color other materials. It is the wrong word to describe the substance administered intravenously during a CT study.[72] That substance is best described as contrast material. Contrast material can indicate the iodinated agents used for CT or the gadolinium-based agents used for MR imaging. Because these agents qualify as a medication, they should be documented in the report not just as "contrast," but with a brand or generic name, a dose, and a route, just like all other medications.

Findings of Doubtful Clinical Significance

The art of being wise is the art of knowing what to overlook.
—William James

One of my most enlightened radiology teachers once told me: "When an experienced radiologist looks at a puzzling finding on an image and doesn't recognize it, it is almost certainly unimportant." We frequently see things on clinical images that we cannot totally explain in terms of known anatomy, physiology, or physics. Yet, there they are. These observations may relate to a little-known or never-before-seen artifact, or perhaps a serendipitous confluence of shadows, or the vestiges of an occult pathophysiologic process. But in each case, they have little bearing on the current health of the patient.

Experienced radiologists know when an observation warrants further work-up and when it does not. They can't always articulate the reason, but they certainly can place a finding beyond the realm of clinical importance. Perhaps this is because experienced radiologists have "seen it all": Anything likely to affect the health of the patient would be recognizable to them. As you gain experience, try describing something you know is unimportant but can't definitively characterize as "findings of doubtful clinical significance." You will avoid the costs of a futile work-up.

Chapter 5:
Mastering Speech Recognition

For a list of all the ways technology has failed to improve the
quality of life, please press three.
—*Alice Kahn*

To radiologists, speech recognition is both an indispensable tool and a vexing time killer. In this chapter, we will focus on understanding and optimizing radiology speech recognition systems.

How Speech Recognition Works

The first step in mastering a speech recognition system is understanding how it works. When I dictate "radiology" into a computer's microphone, the computer receives the sound spectrum shown in Figure 14.

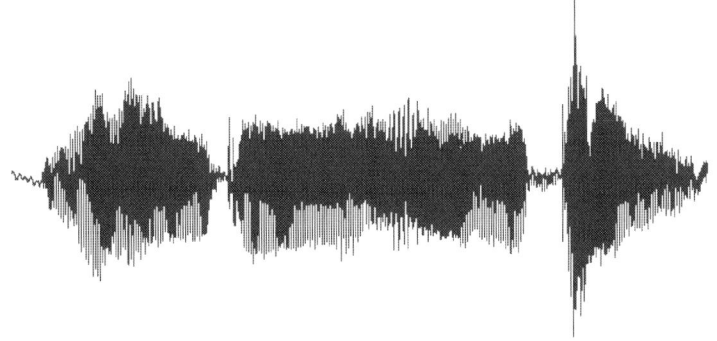

Figure 14. The sound spectrum for the word "radiology."

The computer analyzes this acoustic observation to determine the most common phonemes. *Phonemes* are the smallest unique units of sound from which words are composed. For example, the above spectrum can be divided into nine phonemes: r-a-d-ee-o-l-oh-j-ee. (Note: There are several methods to represent phonemes. I have used WPRK, the Wikipedia pronunciation re-spelling key).[99]

The Acoustic Model and the Language Model

Two distinct mathematical models parse the information in this spectrum. The *acoustic model* manages information about the probability of a word given a series of acoustic observations (i.e., the sounds themselves). Many speech recognition systems include a word-training function that helps you improve the accuracy of the acoustic model for given words. For example, repeatedly pronouncing a word strengthens the computer's linkage of the word to the sequence of phonemes you utter.

Information in the acoustic model is paired with a *language model*, which manages information drawn from typical word sequences in similar narratives (i.e., other radiology reports). The language model estimates the probability of a word given a series of previous words. All modern speech recognition systems use a *tri-gram* language model, meaning they use the previous two words to estimate the probability of the third word. The language model is developed by analyzing a large corpus of text and computing these probabilities in advance. Speech recognition systems could become more accurate by analyzing even longer strings, but current computers are not powerful enough to calculate likelihoods for all the possible four-word combinations in real time.

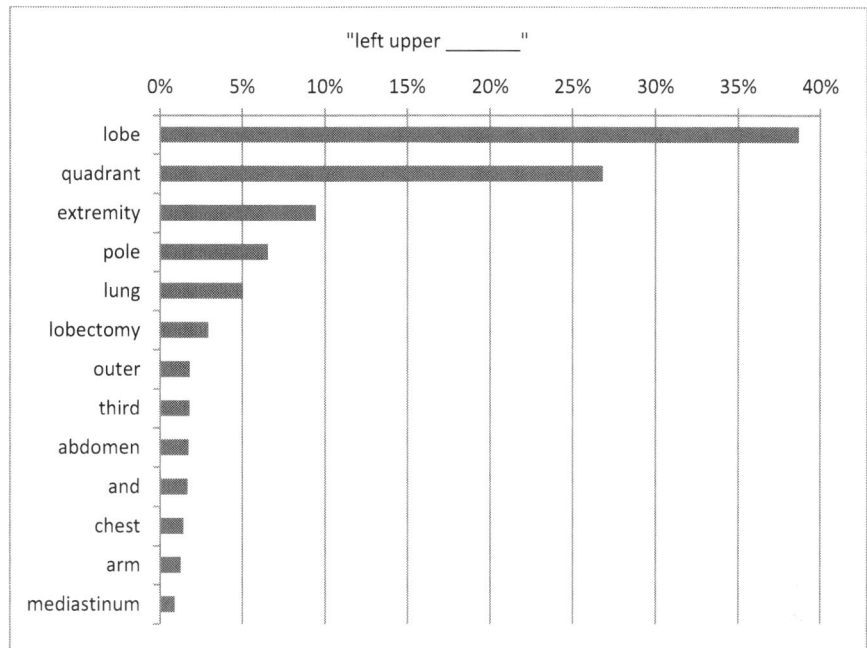

Figure 15. A plot showing the frequency of common tri-grams for "left upper _____" in a large corpus of radiology reports. Tri-grams are powerful tools used by language models to determine the most likely next word.

Figure 15 shows data from a large corpus of radiology reports and illustrates how powerful a language model can be. As we would predict, "left upper lobe" and "left upper quadrant" constitute the majority of three-word combinations beginning with "left upper." This information, even in the absence of any acoustic observations, can yield powerful insights about the likelihood of the next word.

Below is a list of the 10 most common tri-grams in the same corpus of reports:

1. there is no
2. there is a
3. no evidence of
4. of the chest
5. of the right
6. of the left
7. in the right
8. seen in the
9. is no evidence

10. in the left

Here are some other notable tri-grams from the same corpus (with the numbers representing their rank in frequency):

16. within normal limits
29. no active disease
33. heart is normal
34. lungs are clear
46. the prior study
64. left lower lobe
69. the right kidney
80. small amount of
88. a 1.5 Tesla
96. as described above

The Gory Mathematical Details

A more mathematical understanding of speech recognition is shown below. Real-time speech recognition uses a form of Bayesian inference (which we will review in Chapter 10). Expressed mathematically, speech recognition of a single word, W3, looks like this:

$$p(W_3 | O) = \underbrace{p(O | W_3)}_{\substack{\text{Acoustic} \\ \text{model}}} * \underbrace{p(W_3 | W_1 W_2)}_{\substack{\text{Language} \\ \text{model}}},$$

where *p* is the probability function, W1, W2, and W3 are words in sequence, and O is an acoustic observation, or a set of sounds, corresponding to W3. (The vertical bar "|" can be translated as "given.") The equation shows the probability that the next word, W3, is a product of the probability of the acoustic observations given that word (the acoustic model) and the probability of that word given the previous two words (the language model).

Of course, in reality, these systems are much more complex and employ a variety of other optimization methods. The most popular underlying mathematical method is called a *hidden Markov model*. To give you a taste of what is actually going on (and to help you understand why we will not pursue this in greater detail), behold the following excerpt from the Wikipedia entry on speech recognition:[100]

In speech recognition, the hidden Markov model would output a sequence of n-dimensional real-valued vectors (with n being a small integer, such as 10), outputting one of these every 10 milliseconds. The vectors would consist of cepstral coefficients, which are obtained by taking a Fourier transform of a short time window of speech and decorrelating the spectrum using a cosine transform, then taking the first (most significant) coefficients.

Unless you have an advanced degree in mathematics, you're probably as lost as I am. Enough said.

Optimizing Your Speech Recognition

The astounding technologic progress in speech recognition has led to substantial efficiencies in radiology practice. The increasing power of our workstations and the refinement of the statistical techniques used for speech recognition have led to substantial increases in accuracy over the last decade. The accuracy of speech recognition systems in radiology has been measured as high as 98%.

But this new technology also brings new problems: The weaknesses and idiosyncrasies of speech recognition can be the source of endless frustration. Speech recognition accuracy of 98% is still too low. One word in 50 will be incorrect, a 300-word report will contain six errors, and almost all dictated reports will contain at least one error. Many of these errors will remain un-corrected in the final report.[101]

Familiarity with the obscure underlying computational algorithms that drive speech recognition systems can help everyday users understand and manage the behavior (and misbehavior) of these systems. I have been col-lecting speech recognition errors for many years now, and would like to share my collection with you. These errors reveal how speech recognition works (or doesn't work) and often suggest remedies to improve the accuracy of your speech recognition system.

Because speech recognition errors are often humorous, I call them *bloopers*. But as you enjoy the humor, keep in mind that bloopers also can be the source of harmful miscommunications (see Figure 16).

What I Said	What the Computer Wrote
Can't be excluded	Can be excluded
Left basilar atelectasis	Left bacillar atelectasis
1.4 cm	1.47 m
Two days before	Today's before
Discussed by phone	Discussed lipoma
Small amount of pleural fluid	Small bowel pleural fluid
Likely representing lung cancer	Life threatening lung cancer

Figure 16. A sampling of speech recognition errors that may cause harmful miscommunications.

Speech Fail Nonsense

Sometimes the speech recognition system makes mistakes that inadvertently reveal the true idiocy behind its rigid mathematical methods. Figure 17 shows examples of humorous nonsense.

What I Said	What the Computer Wrote
Superior pole of the right kidney	Super Bowl of the right kidney
Morgagni hernia	More gag me hernia
Metacarpophalangeal joint	Metacarpal fail and kill joint
Interphalangeal joints	NFL until joints
Tracheostomy tube	Cake asked me to
A right subclavian PICC terminates	A right suckling and picture mates
Gastroesophageal reflux	Gaseous doctor reflux
Obscures fine detail	Scares fine detail
6:06 a.m.	Success exam
Vasectomy	Visit to me
Bilateral oblique views	Bilateral bleak views

Figure 17. A collection of humorous speech errors. Each of these errors could be avoided if speech recognition systems develop some knowledge about meaning and parts of speech.

Anyone (or any computer) that understood meaning and grammar would never use the word sequences in the second column.

Tip: Remember that speech recognition systems do not perform significant semantic or grammatical analysis. They use a probabilistic approach to determining the next word in a sequence.

Dictionary Bloat

Most speech engines were initially developed for nonmedical applications, such as intelligence gathering and automated phone call management. These general purpose products passed through several corporate hands before emerging as a key medical technology (see Chapter 7). During that transition, there was no incentive to remove words from the dictionary and every reason to add words the system lacked. As a result, speech recognition dictionaries retain many colloquial words that can interfere with good speech recognition but should never appear in a radiology report. A few examples are shown in Figure 18.

What I Said	What the Computer Wrote
Horseshoe kidney	Whores shoes kidney
Thoracolumbar	For rectal lumber
Post-traumatic osteoarthropathy	Poster manic osteoarthropathy
On December 23rd	Undies sever 23rd
Cardiomegaly	Qaeda megaly
2 cm above the carina	To Senate is above the carina
September 2nd	Saddam her second
Tracheostomy tube	Che Cassidy to
Esophagogastric tube	Justice of the vaginal tube
Total knee arthroplasty	Ptolemy arthroplasty
Waxes and wanes	Waxes and Wayne's
February 11th	Farberware 11th

Figure 18. Speech recognition errors that result from words that probably could be removed from the system's vocabulary.

Do we ever need to mention whores, undies, posters, or lumber in our reports? And with all due respect to Ptolemy, Wayne, Che', and Saddam, these proper names also are unnecessary.

Most speech recognition systems provide a mechanism for removing these unwanted words from the dictionary. And many products have already cleaned house since I experienced these errors. But the lesson is clear: When you see an error that produces a word you will never use, delete the word from the system's dictionary to guarantee the error will not recur. Be aggressive in deleting words. In the unlikely event you absolutely need that word in the future, you can always type it. In the extremely unlikely event you frequently need that word, you can always add it back to the system's dictionary.

Tip: When you see a speech recognition error that has produced a word you know you will never use, remove it from the system's dictionary.

Who Is Training Who?

Sometimes, speech recognition systems exhibit a frustrating inability to recognize a word, despite repeated attempts by the user. When this occurs in your reading room, the next sound you may hear will be a microphone (or someone's head) pounding on the desk. Some of my favorite examples are shown in Figure 19.

What I Said	What the Computer Wrote
Mesothelioma	Mesial T. leone
	M(criusic urinoma
	Knees of the ileum
Implantable defibrillator	Implant of the liver for later
	And plantar bleed from a later
	And plentiful do for blader
	Implacable the febrile later
	And plentiful differ but later
	And phleboliths are Berliner
Osteoarthritis	Os urethritis
	*Rightists
	Asterisk redness
	Osseous rites

Figure 19. A collection of recalcitrant speech recognition errors, which could be prevented by intensive system training.

Most systems enable you to "train words" by repeatedly pronouncing the word for the system to hear. As you repeatedly dictate that word, the speech recognition system refines its acoustic model for that word.

Tip: When the system consistently misrecognizes a specific word, train the system more intensively to recognize that word or phrase correctly.

One popular speech recognition engine offers an integrated feature to correct a word or phrase that has been recognized incorrectly. When invoked, a list of its less likely options is displayed, rather like a "differential diagnosis" of this phrase (calculated by the language model). Unfortunately, sometimes the correct answer is not listed, as in this example for "phlebolith" in Figure 20.

Suggestions for "Phlebolith"
Flea bullet
Flee bullet
Flea bulled
Flea Bullit
Flea bullate
Fleet bullet
Flea bulla
Flea bowl with

Figure 20. An unsuccessful use of the "correct that" function for the misrecognition of "phlebolith" in a speech recognition system. The recognition finally improved when I dictated "flab-olith" rather than "fleeb-olith."

Tip: When an error occurs, many systems enable you to correct it from a list of suggestions. This helps improve recognition accuracy in the future and is therefore more effective than simply editing the phrase by hand.

Hearing the proposed remedies for these errors, some may ask, who is training who? Isn't the speech recognition system supposed to modify its behavior in response to our quirks, rather than the other way around? Unfortunately, the current state of technology is too limited to avoid these errors.

Remember the Tri-Gram

Most speech engines are tripped up by short words. Not many words sound like "adenocarcinoma." But plenty of one syllable words containing a long "o" sound can be confused with the word "no." Here are a few examples of short-word bloopers:

What I Said	What the Computer Wrote
Five views	Pi views
The lung is now re-expanded	The lung is not re-expanded
No significant abnormality	Most significant abnormality
Cordis	Coitus
Joints	Giants

Figure 21. Examples of speech recognition errors caused by misrecognition of short words. These errors can be avoided by repeating the word as part of a longer phrase.

Unfortunately, we can't just delete the word "most" from the dictionary to avoid confusion with the word "no." Speaking more clearly and emphasizing the phonetic differences between the two words sometimes can solve this problem. For example, emphasize the "st" sound in "most" and the "d" sound in "Cordis" (or, better yet, substitute the generic word "sheath"). As any frequent user of speech recognition systems knows, changes in pronunciation and diction are sometimes necessary to reduce recurrent errors of this kind.

Another approach leverages the tri-gram. The language model, which calculates the probability of the next word based on the previous two, plays a significant role in good speech recognition. If you redictate only a single word, you lose this accuracy advantage. You will have better luck by repeating a short phrase, which enables the language model and the acoustic model to work together, increasing the chance that the system will get it right the second time around.

Tip: If you encounter an error in a small word, the system is more likely to correct the error if you redictate the entire surrounding phrase, rather than just the small word.

Sound-alikes

A *homophone* is pronounced the same as another word but has a different meaning. For example, "to," "two," and "too" are homophones. Speech recognition systems have difficulty with homophones, for obvious reasons. When a system tries to disambiguate homophones, it must use its language model exclusively because the words sound identical.

What I Said	What the Computer Wrote
C5	Sea 5
Kerley B lines	Curly bee lines
1	One
2	To, two, too,

Figure 22. Examples of speech recognition errors due to words that sound alike. Even the best speech recognition algorithms sometimes have trouble distinguishing between homophones.

A radiologist can do little to improve recognition of homophones, other than to use a language model tailored to radiology. Most speech recognition systems now routinely incorporate radiology-specific language models, and some even develop language models based on reports from your own practice. A more specific language model helps avoid these errors.

Tip: When purchasing a speech recognition system, make sure its language model is specific to radiology.

Date Problems

What I Said	What the Computer Wrote
On April 6th	A nipple sex
December 23rd	These numbers 6th

Figure 23. Examples of speech recognition errors that occur when dictating calendar dates. These can be avoided by dictating dates as numbers separated by slashes or dashes.

Tip: If you are having trouble with dates, trying saying it another way, such as "12 slash 23 slash 2014."

Syllable Emphasis

Some speech recognition errors can be avoided by stressing a different syllable. Figure 24 shows an example.

What I Said	What the Computer Wrote
Interphalangeal	Interfere lunch heel
	NFL until
	Inter fell and she'll
	Inner fail and kill

Figure 24. An example of a speech error that can be avoided by changing the emphasis of syllables in a long word.

Tip: If you are having repetitive problems with a long word, try emphasizing different syllables, such as inter-PHA-lan-GEAL instead of inter-pha-LAN-geal.

Templates and Macros

Template n.: A document or file having a preset format, used as a starting point for a particular application so that the format does not have to be recreated each time it is used.

Macro n.: A single, user-defined command that is part of an application and executes a series of commands

—American Heritage Dictionary

Templates and macros are words or phrases that can be invoked to deposit a larger portion of text into the report. Vendors of speech recognition systems have popularized the term *macro.* But based on the dictionary definitions above, *template* is a more accurate term and is better understood outside the world of radiology reporting. So we will use "template."

Why Templates Matter

Templates save time. Research has repeatedly shown that radiologists who use templates are more efficient than those who report in free text mode.[102] Because templates contain pre-authored text, several advantages accrue to the radiologist: Less cognitive work is required to create and format the report de novo, and less proofreading of the resulting text is needed. Normal and near-normal studies are particularly amenable to templates, with greater gains in time. In many cases, near-normal exams can be reported with a single click or by uttering a single trigger phrase. By investing time in creating speech templates, routine normal reports can be created faster than with conventional dictation.

Templates also improve the reports by making them more complete, with a consistent ordering that helps report readers find information. And because templates can be constructed with consistent text that contains embedded codes, they are more easily processed by a computer. The use of templates also encourages compliance with local or national guidelines and standards, such as the critical test result reporting requirements of the Joint Commission,[103] or the report content measures of the CMS Physician Quality Reporting System (PQRS).[104]

A radiologist reporting in a purely text mode is living in the worst of both worlds. Not only has this radiologist lost the speed advantages to be gained by using templates, but he or she must serve as a clerk and an editor, detecting and correcting speech recognition errors in the text of the report.

Tip: Radiologists who invest in the creation of well-designed templates can improve dictation efficiency.

Template Fields

One of the most powerful features of templates is blanks or *fields*, often delimited by square brackets. Default text may be provided within the field, with an understanding that it may be replaced or modified. Fields enable rapid navigation among parts of the report that are frequently modified (e.g., left/right information) by using the rewind and fast-forward buttons on the microphone to move between fields. Fields also serve as a visual cue for missing information and can signify the availability of other helpful reporting functions, such as a pop-up list of predetermined choices to fill in a field.

Template Reporting Styles

Radiologists tend to employ templates in several different ways. One of the most common reporting modes uses a single template to serve as a blueprint for the entire report. Some reporting systems insert this initial template automatically, or they offer a short list of template choices, based on the exam code, the imaging modality, or the body part being imaged. Once an initial template is selected, it is typically presented to the radiologist using a text-editor metaphor, similar to Microsoft Word. Thus, the radiologist can use an initial template to guide interaction with the reporting system to create a report by filling in fields.

More sophisticated users of reporting systems will use not only a default template, but also additional smaller templates to "fill in the blanks" as part of a nested assembly process. Some systems provide trigger words for each choice on a pick list, allowing fields to be filled by using microphone commands rather than the mouse. For example, the radiologist may begin with an overall template containing fields, filling each field by uttering a trigger word that inserts a specific phrase.

A third style of reporting, used by a only small minority of radiologists, employs a large set of small templates, each of which contains a phrase or short sentence related to the report, such as atelectasis, a central line, or a normal heart. These templates generally do not contain blanks that need to be filled and are assembled in series to create a report. This approach requires significant forethought to ensure the templates are strung together to produce well-formatted reports.

The optimal reporting style depends not only on the proclivities of the radiologist, but also on the type of study being reported. For example, serial assembly is more often used to report a chest radiograph study performed in the ICU; in this context, there are a large number of brief elements (e.g., the position of tubes and lines) that must be assembled in multiple combinations. Creating a new template for each combination of observations would require an intractable explosion of phrase sequences.

Fill-in-the-blanks mode works well for radiologists who are less sophisticated users, but nevertheless want consistent ordering of content and are willing to fill in each field with narrative. Nested assembly works well for sophisticated users who report complex studies and can give substantial advanced consideration to the design of their templates and how they will be used in combination.

Tip: For maximum reporting speed, use nested assembly of short templates to fill in the blanks of a detailed initial template. Time invested in the creation of such an integrated system of templates is well spent.

Speech Recognition: A Critical Analysis

I first realized that speech recognition had become entrenched in my practice when I received a call from a referring clinician who was mildly perturbed that he had not yet received the report for one of his patients. I asked him when the images became available, and he replied "about 10 minutes ago."

In days gone by, a 12-hour report turnaround time was considered progress[105] because transcription was performed in batches. But today, the transcription signature queue no longer delays the referring clinician's receipt of the report. Once speech recognition is implemented, transcription delays disappear for reports dictated by the attending radiologist because they are signed immediately. As speech recognition raised the bar for report turnaround time, customer expectations followed.

Improved report turnaround also can reduce reimbursement delays for the study, improving a practice's bottom line. So speech recognition can improve both customer service and financial performance.

The following sections cover additional strengths and weaknesses of using speech recognition systems.

Transcription Is Error Prone, Too

In our frustration with speech recognition errors, we sometimes forget that transcriptionists make mistakes. One study found that 33.8% of reports required post-transcription editing by radiologists prior to signature.[106] Nearly 6% of the corrected errors were substantive, such as errors of missing or incorrect information that would have led to unnecessary treatment or testing or that could have caused risk of complications or morbidity for the patient.

Return on Investment

Speech recognition saves money. Transcription services are a costly recurring expense. Transcription services can drain 2%–5% of practice revenues. Speech recognition systems often cost as much as 1–2 years of transcription services but permanently eliminate transcription expenses from the operating budget. Alternatively, speech recognition systems can be purchased as an operating expense, similar to transcription services, but at a fraction of the cost. Whether the hospital or the radiology practice pays for transcription, there is a strong financial incentive to adopt speech recognition.

The Radiologist as Editor

Unfortunately, radiologists are not the main financial beneficiaries of adopting speech recognition systems. Practice managers improve their bottom lines and referring providers benefit from faster turnaround of reports. But the radiologists who use the system typically derive little or no financial benefit, unless they are owners of a radiology practice that itself is paying for transcription.

Use of speech recognition systems has substantial hidden costs for the radiologists. Error rates have been improving and are now likely closer to 100% than 95%. Nevertheless, errors will appear in the typical radiology report. The costs of error correction don't show up explicitly on the bottom line, but can be a serious drag on productivity, and therefore on the finances of a practice. The proofreader is not a transcriptionist being paid $12 per hour, but a radiologist earning many times that. Many radiologists rightly believe this work is not a productive use of their time. Add a half a minute to the time to finalize more than a hundred reports a radiologist dictates in a day, and that radiologist will be leaving for home an hour later each evening. This situation is not a prescription for a happy work environment.

Tip: As you analyze the financial effects of using speech recognition systems, consider the hidden editing costs.

The Correctionist Model

Some radiologists feel that the "correctionist model," in which speech recognition is used to create reports that are then sent to transcriptionists to correct, represents a happy medium. But this approach marries the disadvantages of speech recognition (fumbling with technology, look-away time) with the disadvantages of transcription (cost, delays in report turnaround). The correctionist model can serve as a temporary transitional model for radiologists who are particularly resistant to weaning from transcription. But only a practice with deep pockets and a strong hold on its referral base should use this as a permanent solution.

Factors Leading to Successful Adoption

I was a young attending radiologist when speech recognition was first adopted by my practice in 2000. And I have since led a large practice through two speech recognition vendor changes and ran a startup that became a speech recognition vendor. As a grizzled combat veteran of the speech recognition "wars," I have two pieces advice: one serious and one tongue-in-cheek. The serious advice: Users' responses to change can be dramatically different. Some individuals will love a new system, some will dislike it intensely, and most will be willing to come along for the ride.[107] These reactions are particularly true for adoption of speech recognition systems, which perform differently for each user based on voice timbre, elocution accuracy, ambient noise in the reading room, and numerous other factors. Figure 25 illustrates the spectrum of responses to these new systems.

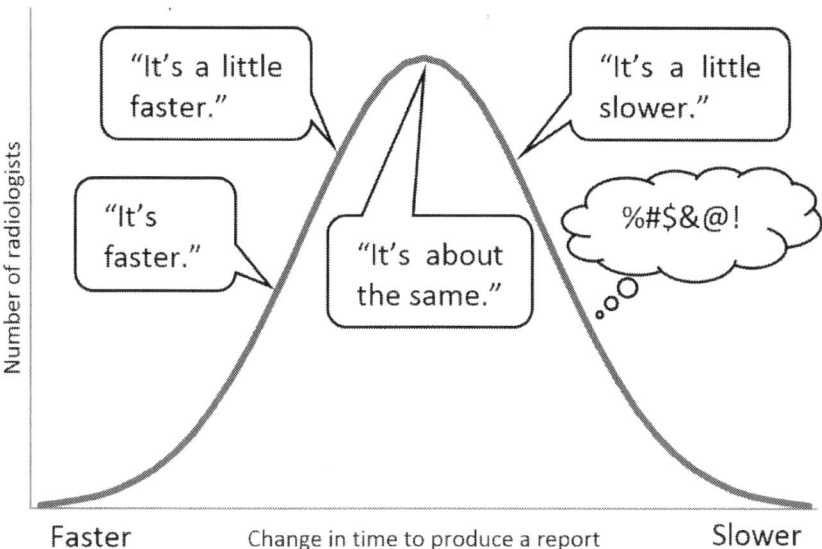

Figure 25. The diversity of radiologists' reactions to a new speech recognition system.

My tongue-in-cheek advice on speech recognition adoption is expressed as a riddle. Question: How do you make radiologists like the speech recognition system they are currently using? Answer: Replace it with a new one. Speech recognition products are probabilistic, inherently imperfect, and occasionally frustrating. The grass often seems greener on the other side of the fence, whether considering "good old" methods or the "perfectly accurate" system used by a colleague in another practice.

Despite these pros and cons of speech recognition, there is one unavoidable truth: There is no going back.

Chapter 6:
Organizing the Radiology Report

A basic structural design underlies every kind of writing.
—William Strunk and E.B. White, The Elements of Style[71]

If you ask radiologists today whether they think standardization of reports is a good idea, most agree.[24,108] The core elements of the report are quite similar across radiology practices. For years, radiologists have advocated a standard organization of report elements.[30] Yet, reaching consensus on a standard remains elusive for many radiology practices, perhaps because radiologists worry that a standard may rob them of their favorite phrase or format when their style differs from that of their colleagues.

Agreeing on common section headings across a practice can be a less controversial starting point for standardization. The RSNA Reporting Committee recognized this common entry point to standardization and created a valuable resource for those wanting to get started. What follows is a review of RSNA's consensus "master report template" (with a few minor modifications) that emerged from a forum in 2008.[109] Similar standard headings have been advocated by others.[13,110] If all radiologists adhere to these principles of report structure and content, reports will be easier to read, communication will be clearer, and patients will be safer.

Patient Identifiers

More than once, I have dictated a report into the wrong patient's medical record. Here is how it happened: I launched the images and report for Mrs.

Jones. A referring clinician's phone call interrupted me with a request to review the images on Mr. Smith, which I quickly launched on my PACS (picture archiving and communication system) workstation. Once I completed my review of Mr. Smith's images, I decided to dictate Mr. Smith's report while my observations were fresh in my mind. Failing to notice that the reporting system was still waiting for the report on Mrs. Jones, I dictated Mr. Smith's report into Mrs. Jones's medical record.

Misfiled radiology reports are a pervasive problem.[111] Definitive identification of the patient to which a report belongs is an essential element of patient safety. In the past, the radiologist might write the patient's name on the report or dictate the name and an identifier into a recording system. In the more recent past, bar-coding systems were used to automate accurate patient identification. Problems with patient identification abate as electronic work lists and integrated computer systems ensure that the patient shown in the reporting system matches the patient in the displayed images at all times. And most imaging devices now can receive a standard work list that contains the scheduled patients for the day.[112] The technologist creating the images chooses the patient from a list of the day's orders, eliminating the possibility of typographic errors.

Tip: Systems that require manual entry of the accession number, or that don't maintain synchrony between systems, can cause misidentification errors. Select a single system to drive radiologist work flow that launches all other systems in the correct patient context.

Clinical History

The Clinical History section describes the reason for the exam and other patient history relevant to the interpretation of the study. A diagnosis code often is provided to ensure medical necessity for billing purposes. Ideally, the referring clinician should transmit this information with the request. Overwhelming evidence shows that a detailed clinical history improves radiologists' accuracy in detecting and characterizing abnormalities.[113–124] Many radiologists are taught that the images should be reviewed both before and after reading the clinical history to avoid bias.[125]

The electronic medical record (EMR) represents a rich source of clinical information for the radiologist.[126] But at most institutions, radiologists do not yet have ready access to the EMR. Paradoxically, the advent of information technology to store the patient's medical records has on average reduced the information available to the radiologist.[127,128] EMR systems typically require a separate sign-on, a manual search for the patient at hand, and substantial time sifting through the electronic chart to find data relevant to the radiology study at hand. Some institutions are designing radiology-tailored views into their EMR systems, but these tools are still uncommon. Many other organizations are transitioning to radiology information systems (RISs) that are embedded in the EMR. Until radiology systems are tightly interconnected to other clinical information systems, many radiologists will lack ready access to detailed clinical information.

Radiologists are in the dark for another reason: Because reports and the associated images are distributed electronically to the EMR system, referring clinicians obtain the imaging information they need without leaving their offices. They have little need to visit the radiology reading room, where in the past they might have given the radiologist rich clinical history and follow-up.

Some reporting systems insert a brief clinical history automatically into a field in the report template. If the inserted history is correct and sufficient for medical necessity, there is no need for the radiologist to dictate it again, with one exception: when the radiologist wants to demonstrate awareness of the history at the time of interpretation. For example, the referring clinician should be aware that you knew the patient's immune system was compromised when you interpreted the chest radiograph.

Clinical history provides a reason for performing the study, which is required for reimbursement. "Rule out" histories are insufficient for most health care payers. Instead, the clinical history should provide a symptom-based reason for the study. For example, "fever, cough" is a reimbursable history for a chest radiograph study, whereas "r/o pneumonia" by itself is not. If no relevant history is provided, abnormalities discovered by the radiologist can be used to justify the medical necessity of the exam. But if no history or observations document medical necessity, the radiology practice must contact the referring provider to find the reason for the exam and document it in the radiology report.

Tip: Detailed clinical history improves the interpretation accuracy of radiologists. Reports must contain sufficient clinical history to justify the performance of the study. Templates with prefilled fields can facilitate this documentation.

Imaging Technique

The Technique section of the report describes how the images were acquired. This section interests radiologists more than anyone else. When dictating this section, keep in mind this question: If you were interpreting the follow-up study, what would you want to know? Most radiologists appreciate knowing the patient's position, the imaging modality, and any special coils, transducers, or other ancillary equipment that was employed. The basic technical specifications of the imaging device are helpful, including device configuration, and the imaging sequences that were acquired. Figure 26 lists key Technique items valued by radiologists.

The Joint Commission, a ubiquitous hospital certification body, requires that all medications administered to the patient must be documented in the patient's medical record; contrast agents are no exception. Therefore, oral and intravenous contrast material (and any other medications) administered during a radiologic examination should be documented using medication name, dose, and route of administration (e.g., "Midazolam 1 mg IV"). Some reporting systems allow this information to be imported automatically into a template field.

Health care payers also pay close attention to the Technique section. As a result, there is a risk of revenue loss if critical information is inadvertently omitted from this section of the report. To be reimbursed at a higher rate, certain exams require specific documentation of imaging technique. The most commonly omitted elements are documentation of intravenous contrast administration, the number of views obtained for radiographic studies, and organs visualized during abdominal ultrasound studies. If you want to get full payment for performing and interpreting the study, include the required elements.

Tip: Some reporting systems import medication information automatically into the radiology report. This feature boosts reporting efficiency, avoids redictation errors, and ensures complete documentation.

Modality	Technique Suggestions
Radiography	Body part imaged
	Number of views, type of view if clinically relevant
Fluoroscopy	Body region imaged
	Oral contrast agent administered
	Glucagon or other medications administered
	Fluoroscopy time
CT	Craniocaudal range of imaging
	Intravenous and oral contrast agents administered
	Imaging planes, if clinically relevant
	Any special formatting or reconstruction performed
	Phase of enhancement, if applicable
MR imaging	Body region imaged
	Magnetic field strength and coils used, if applicable
	Intravenous and oral contrast agents administered
	Imaging planes, if clinically relevant
	Brief pulse sequence descriptions
	Any special formatting or reconstruction performed
	Phase of enhancement, if applicable
Ultrasound	Structures imaged or attempted
	Study complexity (e.g., complete or limited), if applicable
	Mode (e.g., Doppler), if applicable
	Special transducers (e.g., transvaginal), if applicable
	Intravenous contrast agent administered
	Patient maneuvers (e.g., Valsalva), if applicable
Nuclear and molecular imaging	Body region imaged
	Radiopharmaceuticals and other medications administered
	Image acquisition views and sequences
Interventional	Sterile preparation, if applicable
	Description of the procedure itself
	Fluoroscopy time and radiation dose information
	Contrast agent and other medications administered
	Specimens sent to pathology, if applicable
	Complications, if applicable
	Attending radiologist who supervised, if performed with trainee

Figure 26. Key items to report in the Technique section for various modalities.

Image Quality

The radiology report should describe any limitations of the study that interfere with accurate interpretation. Image quality information often is included in the Technique section, since most image quality issues relate directly to how the images were acquired. If the study is limited, a reason should be provided, such as the patient's inability to cooperate, suboptimal positioning, or other factors. Some studies require an explicit recounting of how the limitations hamper the ability to draw conclusions from the study,[129] but in most cases, the statement should be brief and need not describe every detail that did not go according to plan.[12,130]

A crucial quality decision is whether the study is sufficiently degraded to warrant repetition of the exam. This decision requires clinical judgment—there are no hard and fast rules. The key factor is whether the clinical question can be answered by the images. For example, when a preoperative chest radiograph of a healthy middle-aged patient undergoing cataract surgery fails to show a few millimeters of one lung apex, I will comment on it only briefly and let it pass. On the other hand, if the same limitation is present on a study obtained to determine whether pneumothorax is present, I consider the exam non-diagnostic and recommend that the view be repeated. Many practices will offer such a repeat study at no charge, particularly when the cause of the limitation was a shortcoming of radiology quality control.

Tip: As radiology reports are increasingly viewed by patients in online patient portals, it is more important than ever to avoid language that appears to blame the patient for problems. A patient may be unable to follow instructions for a variety of reasons, including concurrent illness, mobility difficulties, stress, or various forms of mental impairment. Patients who do not cooperate well with imaging protocols are usually *unable* to cooperate, rather than unwilling.

Comparison Exams

The American College of Radiology (ACR) guideline for communication of diagnostic imaging findings[131] states "Comparisons with previous examinations and reports, when possible, are a part of the radiologic consultation and report." Radiologists must determine whether relevant prior exams are available, whether through the RIS, PACS, or speech recognition system. And each report should contain a section devoted to listing the previous images or reports to which the current examination was compared.

Comparison with previous exams is a wise choice. Referring to comparisons significantly improves the accuracy of radiologic interpretation and can save the radiologist from embarrassing and costly errors.[132,133] Comparison exams can obviate additional imaging.[134] Comparison with prior studies is essential when there is an abnormality to follow or when additional clinical history is needed.[135] Because interobserver variability among radiologists is common,[136,137] review of prior reports can avoid embarrassing inconsistencies among radiologists. The prior report can also serve as an important risk management tool.[138] Reading the interpretation of another radiologist who has viewed the prior images, which are often quite similar to the current study, is a learning tool for trainees. Prior reports are readily available in most modern systems, so take a look.

Tip: Unless you need to indicate you compared a specific image, use *relative dates* to indicate when comparison exams were reported. The concept of "1 week ago" is more easily understood by report readers than computing the number of days between March 5, 2008 and February 27, 2008. When imaging occurs at a regular frequency (e.g., daily in the ICU), relative dates (e.g., "yesterday") also expedite the use of a previous report as a template for the current one, a popular feature available in some reporting systems.

Findings or Observations

All we want are the facts, ma'am.
—*Sergeant Joe Friday, Dragnet*

The Findings section is the heart of the radiology report, where the imaging observations are described, sentence by sentence. We reviewed in detail how these sentences should be created in Chapters 2 through 4. The Findings section should contain factual descriptions of what is observed, along with expressions of size, severity, and uncertainty about those observations. The ideal radiology report will contain a series of brief declarative sentences in the present tense, such as "The ventricles are normal in size, shape, and position." When the story of how specific findings (e.g., blunting of the costophrenic angle) relate to a pathophysiologic process (e.g., a pleural effusion) or a clinical diagnosis (e.g., congestive heart failure) is complex, the Findings section should provide the necessary rhetorical support.

Summary or Impression

*When you have written your headline, you have spent eighty
cents out of your dollar.*
—David Ogilvy

The Summary section is of paramount importance, since many referring clinicians read only this section.[20,42,139] The Summary should list the most important conclusions that can be drawn from the imaging observations and the clinical history. The salient observations should be listed in order of importance. Any query posed by the referring clinician should be answered. Recommendations for additional imaging or other follow-up should be listed, if applicable.

A few additional items should be included in or near the Summary, owing to their importance for continuity of care and clarity of communication. For example, the Joint Commission requires documented notification of unexpected or critical test results. This record is best placed in the Summary.

More and more states, and some federal financial incentives, require documentation of radiation exposure in the report—another item that fits nicely in the Summary section. Global assessment codes, such as the BI-RADS assessment categories for breast imaging and increasingly similar scales for other types of examinations,[140–144] are best placed in the Summary as well.

The naming of this section generates mild controversy. In the distant past, the final section of the report has been called "Conclusion" or the even bolder "Diagnosis."[30,145] However, a recent consensus statement recommended either "Impression" or "Summary".[109] About half of radiologists, myself included, prefer to call it the "Impression" section, although that term is becoming less common. Many radiologists call it the "Summary," clearly conveying this section's role as an authoritative listing of the significant observations. Whatever your preference, you should choose one of these designations—either Impression or Summary— and use it consistently across your practice.

Some radiologists believe that only specific statements of fact belong in the Findings section and that linkage between findings, logical inferences, and diagnostic conclusions should be reserved for the Summary section. That approach sometimes leads to a long narrative Summary that may obfuscate findings of high clinical significance. The alternative view (which I favor) is that the Summary should contain a prioritized list of the clinically relevant and actionable findings—a brief recapitulation of key elements of the Findings section. Although the merit of this format has not been studied directly, I suspect that many busy referring clinicians appreciate its brevity and focus.

Standard Report Elements: A Reference Guide

Here is a brief summary of the report elements described above:
Patient Identifiers
- Ensure that the report is associated with the correct patient.
- List age and gender for clinical context.

Clinical History
- Describe reason for the exam, including medical necessity.
- List specific questions posed by the referring clinician.

Comparison
- Include the date and type of any comparison images or reports.

Imaging Technique
- Identify the imaging device and its configuration.
- Briefly describe patient positioning and any diagnostic maneuvers.
- Document any medications administered, including contrast material.
- Describe any limitations of image quality.

Findings or Observations
- Use short declarative sentences to describe what the images show (see Chapters 2 through 4.)

Summary or Impression
- List all clinically significant findings in order of importance.
- Include any resulting recommendations.

Part II:
History and Foundations

Chapter 7:
The History of Radiology Reporting

Most of the things worth doing in the world had been declared impossible before they were done.
—*Louis D. Brandeis*

When I began radiology training in 1990, my department had just implemented one of the first radiology information systems (RISs). It tracked the location of film jackets and managed the schedule for each of our imaging devices. When the patient arrived, a card was printed to identify the patient, the scheduled study, and a few words of clinical information. Images were created on film and attached to the card with a paper clip. When the study was complete, films were brought to the reading room and hung on light boxes or film alternators (a big motorized device with rotating lighted panels controlled by foot pedals), usually by an aide or a resident.

My department was in the midst of a transition from an older phone-based transcription system to cassette tapes, which recorded all the dictations from each area. Cassette recorders with microphones attached were available at each film alternator. Members of the transcription pool circulated frequently to collect the tapes and bring us new ones. Back in the transcription pool, they listened to the tapes and transcribed the reports into the new RIS. Everyone checked the RIS periodically to see whether new reports were available for electronic editing and signature.

I still remember the anguished cries of some senior radiologists for whom the RIS was the first encounter with a keyboard of any kind. Radiologists were slow to sign their reports. Even with this relatively efficient (for its day) system, often more than 24 hours elapsed before reports were available. A day or two more elapsed before printed versions were filed in the paper hospital chart or mailed to the referring physician (with a stamp!). These delays were not unique to our radiology practice.[105]

Since those days, radiology work is increasingly automated, bringing unimagined efficiencies but also new problems. We now display digital images on picture archiving and communication systems (PACS), eliminating the cost of the films and the need for the aide who hung them. Our RIS now tracks the myriad milestones of the patient experience, from scheduling to check-in to exam completion and finalization. And because of a powerful new work list standard (courtesy of DICOM [Digital Imaging and Communications in Medicine]),[112] when a patient arrives in our department, his or her name can be selected on the console of the imaging device, obviating the need for the technologist to retype (or mistype) the patient information. Once the images are acquired, they are launched immediately from work lists available to all radiologists throughout our practice. Any study is displayed by the PACS in less than a second. Cross-sectional images are viewed in cine mode on a computer monitor, rather than on eight film panels, each containing 15 miniscule images. When the study is launched, comparison images are displayed automatically, and the reporting system opens in context. For some practices, the electronic medical record (EMR) displays a succinct summary of the patient.[126] The radiologist uses a speech recognition system to create, edit, and sign the report in real time. The final report is available to providers everywhere just minutes after the study is complete.

These striking changes have profoundly affected the practice of radiology over the last 25 years. In the sections that follow, we will reach even further back into history to understand the potent influences on radiology reporting over an even longer arc of time, with equally dramatic consequences.

The Narrative Report

Since the advent of the x-ray, radiology reporting tools have moved from the inkwell to the cassette tape to the computer microphone. And the focus of report creation has traveled from the radiologist to the transcriptionist and back again. But even as we have adopted electronic reporting systems, the overall metaphor for interacting with the report is that of a text editor with an insertion point—the same metaphor used by the word processing software we use to prepare other documents. Radiologists have free reign to examine the images and create a narrative that captures the findings and their implications, unconstrained by standards for nomenclature or format. It is not surprising that variety abounds.

Today's narrative reports also are subtly constrained by the information systems in which they are created. Most interfaces that transmit radiology reports see them as a collection of unformatted characters, to be ingested and spit out in a linear fashion. Font sizes, boldface, and italic type, which are the mainstay of even the most rudimentary word processing programs, are not retained. So reports UPPER CASE for section headings and blank lines to separate paragraphs often are the only formatting tools available.

Some modern information systems add seemingly personal but ironically robotic elements to narrative radiology reports, such as a salutation at the beginning—"Dear Dr. Smith, Thank you for referring this patient to me"—and a cheery sign-off at the end—"If you have any questions, please feel free to call me. Best regards, Dr. Mary Jones." These perfunctory greetings paradoxically resemble the collegial service-oriented attitude embodied by Dr. Morton's letter, but they lose much of their meaning through rote repetition.

Narrative reporting has persisted over the decades because of its efficiency for radiologists and became intrinsic to the dictation systems that arose during the same era. Dictating is efficient because the radiologist's eyes remain on the images. Dictation requires little training. There is no need to forge a consensus on terminology and format. In short, narrative reports have evolved for the convenience of the report author, not the report reader. As radiologists face pressures to demonstrate their tangible value to patient care, radiologists' reporting styles must adapt to the needs of their customers: referring clinicians and patients.

How did we arrive at these current reporting practices, which are almost exclusively narrative? And how should we respond to the pressures to change our methods? Before we answer these questions, we will review several unique historical reporting methods that will help us understand important context.

Anatomic Diagrams

We may now look where we have previously only been able to listen.
—*Francis Henry Williams, MD* [146]

The use of icons, sketches, and other visual representations to report imaging findings has since been advocated by many radiologists. [147] Around the turn of the 20th century, this nonnarrative form of early reporting was advocated by Francis Henry Williams, a renowned physician at Boston City Hospital who had obtained an engineering degree from Massachusetts Institute of Technology before becoming a physician.[148]

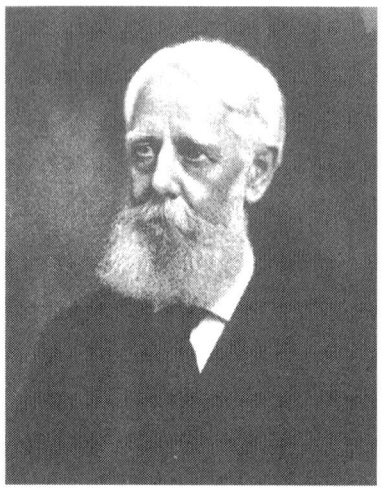

Figure 27. Dr. Francis Henry Williams in 1924.[146]

Dr. Williams's early reports were anatomic line drawings on which he sketched pathologic conditions.

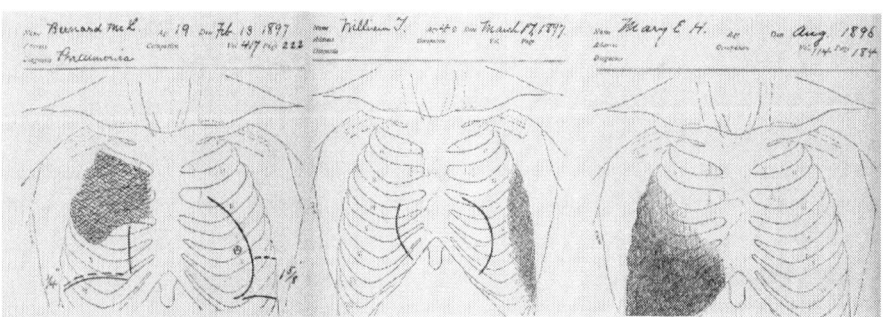

Figure 28. Dr. Francis Henry Williams's early anatomic sketches depicting, from left to right, right upper lobe pneumonia, pleurisy with effusion, and encysted pleurisy. Figures 106, 130, and 136 in reference [149].

Nearly a century later, radiology researchers in Goteborg, Sweden, developed a radiology reporting system called MEDELA based on typing numbers into a computer terminal. The numbers were specified by graphical forms.

Figure 29 shows an example of one such form for the hypopharynx, esophagus, and gastric cardia.[150]

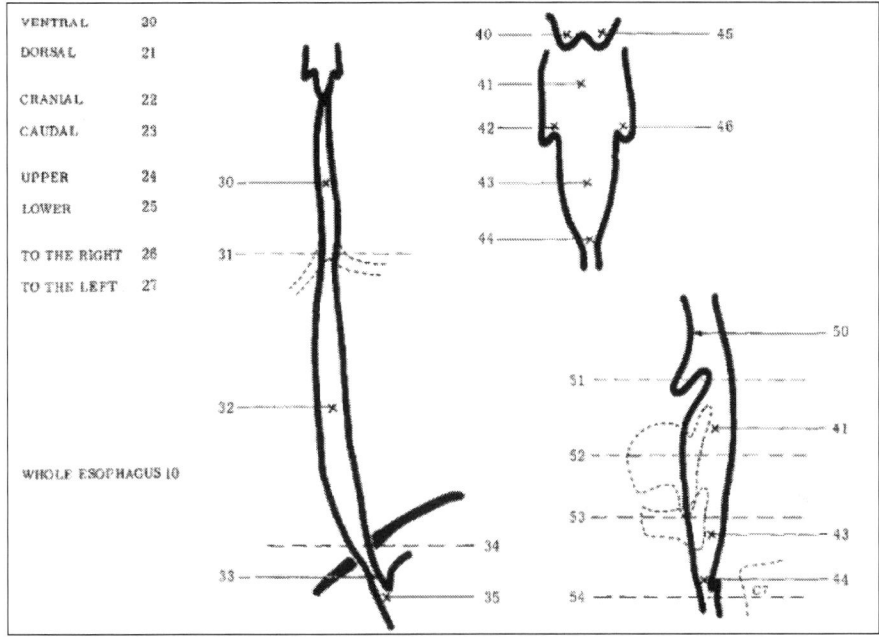

Figure 29. A graphical form indicating the appropriate number
to record in a computer terminal to create a radiology report.[150]
(Reproduced with permission from Brolin, I. MEDELA: An
Electronic Data-Processing System for Radiological Reporting.
Radiology 103, 249–255, 1972. Copyright RSNA.)

Well into the 20th century, radiologists considered that marking areas of suspicion with arrows constituted a sufficient radiology report.[151] As new technologies and user interfaces enable rapid creation of multimedia reports, these innovative diagrams from the MEDELA system can serve as early models for the visual reporting of clinical imaging findings.[152,153]

Handwritten Checklists

Roentgenology is and of right ought to be, a legitimate specialty.
—*Russell D. Carman, MD*

Dr. Russell Carman, another early radiology pioneer who established the radiology department at the Mayo Clinic in 1913,[154] advocated the use of checklists or templates, filled in with multiple-choice responses and hand-written observations. These printed sheets were quickly completed by circling an appropriate response or filling in a blank.

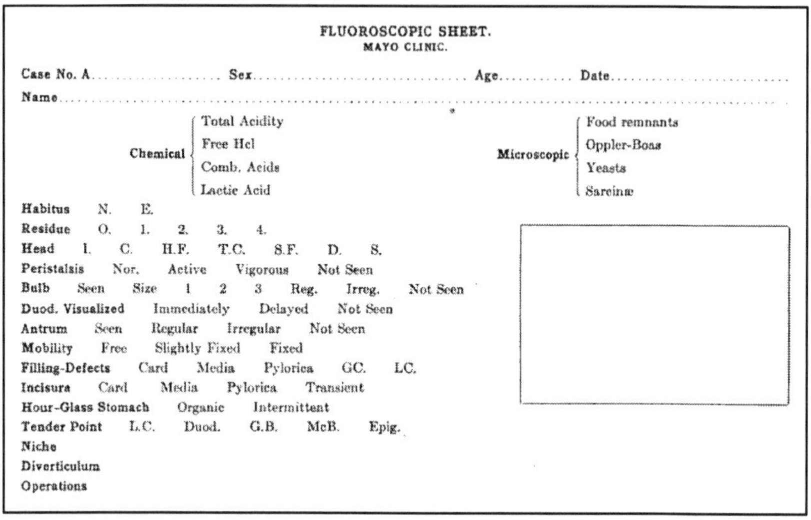

FLUOROSCOPIC SHEET.
MAYO CLINIC.

Case No. A.................. Sex.............................. Age.......... Date........................
Name..

Chemical: Total Acidity; Free Hcl; Comb. Acids; Lactic Acid
Microscopic: Food remnants; Oppler-Boas; Yeasts; Sarcinæ

Habitus N. E.
Residue O. 1. 2. 3. 4.
Head 1. C. H.F. T.C. S.F. D. S.
Peristalsis Nor. Active Vigorous Not Seen
Bulb Seen Size 1 2 3 Reg. Irreg. Not Seen
Duod. Visualized Immediately Delayed Not Seen
Antrum Seen Regular Irregular Not Seen
Mobility Free Slightly Fixed Fixed
Filling-Defects Card Media Pylorica GC. LC.
Incisura Card Media Pylorica Transient
Hour-Glass Stomach Organic Intermittent
Tender Point L.C. Duod. G.B. McB. Epig.
Niche
Diverticulum
Operations

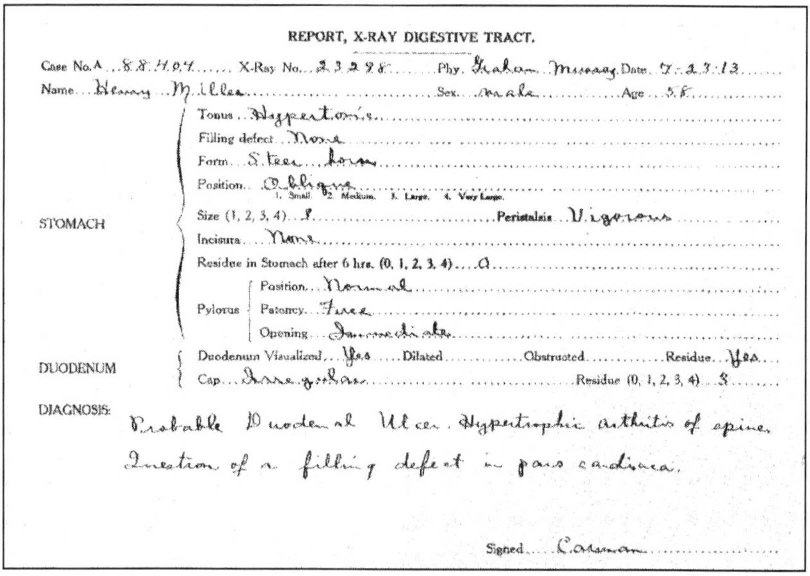

REPORT, X-RAY DIGESTIVE TRACT.

Case No. A ..88404...... X-Ray No...23298...... Phy. Graham Murray Date 7-23-13......
Name... Henry Miller........................ Sex. male........... Age...58.............

STOMACH
Tonus.. Hypertonic..
Filling defect.. None..
Form... Steer horn..
Position... Oblique..
1. Small. 2. Medium. 3. Large. 4. Very Large.
Size (1, 2, 3, 4)... 2......................... Peristalsis Vigorous..............
Incisura.... None..
Residue in Stomach after 6 hrs. (0, 1, 2, 3, 4).... 0..
Pylorus: Position... Normal.......................; Patency... Free.......................; Opening... Immediate.......................

DUODENUM
Duodenum Visualized... Yes..... Dilated............ Obstructed............ Residue... Yes...
Cap... Irregular.................................... Residue (0, 1, 2, 3, 4)... 3........

DIAGNOSIS: Probable Duodenal Ulcer. Hypertrophic arthritis of spine. Question of a filling defect in pars cardiaca.

Signed..... Carman....................

Figure 30. One of Dr. Russell Carman's early template reports. Top: Figure 2 in reference [155]. Bottom: Page 748 in reference [4]. More examples in reference [156].

These simple visual and structured reports did not catch on at the time, probably because imaging became more complex, and reporting speed became an imperative. Conventional dictation remained the dominant form of radiology reporting in the early 20th century.

Computer-based Reporting

I think there is a world market for maybe five computers.
—*Thomas J. Watson*

Sixty years later, well before the advent of automated speech recognition, it became feasible to use computers in a clinical setting. Almost immediately, radiologists began to reexamine the use of electronic checklists and multimedia to capture report information from radiologists.

Despite the limited computers of the late 1960s and the 1970s, that era became a heyday for the development of new reporting systems. Henry Pendergrass and colleagues from the Massachusetts General Hospital developed a system that created a report through a branching question-and-answer dialogue.[157] This system ran on a Digital Equipment Corporation PDP-7 computer, which was considered cheap and powerful for its time. The computer had 144 Kbytes of memory and a 250-KHz processor speed (all for the low, low price of about $72,000.) Around the same time, Robert Greenes, a radiologist and one of Pendergrass's collaborators, described a similar experimental system for medical progress notes in the *New England Journal of Medicine*.[158]

Alphanumeric Codes

Beth Israel Hospital in Boston developed the Coded Language Information Processing (CLIP) system in the mid 1970s. Letter and number codes typed on a keyboard were used to enter a report into CLIP. Figure 31 shows the "easily memorized" alphabetic coding system, part of a larger branching tree structure. For example, *R5/M1S1;N21* can be decoded as follows: *R5* for the *Respiratory system, lung parenchyma*; *M1* for a *Mass lesion, solid*; *S1* for *Shape, rounded*; *N21* for *Neoplasm, primary malignant, carcinoma*.

: ANATOMY	/ FINDINGS	; ETIOLOGY
A ANATOMIC AREA	A ALL NORMAL	A ALL NORMAL
B BONE	B BREACH OF STRUCTURE	B BACTERIAL OR OTHER BUG
C CARDIAC	C CALCULUS OR FOREIGN BODY	C CONGENITAL OR DEVELOPMEN-TAL
D DIGESTIVE	D DEVITALIZED OR DEAD TISSUE, ULCER	D DEGENERATIVE
E ENDOCRINE	E —EDGE CHARACTERISTIC	E ENDOCRINE DISORDER
F FUNCTIONAL BODY SPACE	F FREE FLUID OR GAS	F FEEDING DISORDER
G GENITAL	G+ —GRADE OF SEVERITY OR STAGE	G+ —GRADE OF SEVERITY OR STAGE
H HEMATIC	H* HYDRODYNAMIC DISTURBANCE	H HEMATOLOGIC DISORDER
I INTEGUMENTARY & BREAST	I INFILTRATION OR CONSOLIDA-TION	I IMMUNOLOGIC OR INFLAMMA-TORY
J JOINT	J —JUDGE FINDINGS	J —JUDGE DIAGNOSIS
K —KEY PHRASE OR WORD	K —KEY PHRASE OR WORD	K —KEY PHRASE OR WORD
L LYMPHATIC	L LUMEN DEFORMITY	L —LIBRARY, TEACHING, RESEARCH
M MUSCULAR	M MASS LESION	M METABOLIC DISORDER
N NERVOUS	N* NEUROMUSCULAR DYSFUNCTION	N NEOPLASTIC OR DYSPLASTIC
P PREGNANCY	P —POSITION OR DISPLACEMENT	P PSYCHIATRIC
Q+ —QUANTITY	Q+ —QUANTITY: SIZE, NUMBER, RATE	Q+ —QUANTITY
R RESPIRATORY	R REPAIR OR FIBROSIS	R REACTION: DRUG, DUST, CHEMI-CAL
S —SIDE SIGHT & SOUND	S —SHAPE OR DEFORMATION	S SURGICAL
T TEETH	T —TEXTURE OR TISSUE DERANGE-MENT	T TRAUMATIC
U URINARY	U —UPDATED FINDINGS	U UNKNOWN, BUT DIAGNOSTIC
V VASCULAR	V* VISCERAL DYSFUNCTION	V VASCULAR DISORDER
W —WHEREABOUT?	W —WHEREABOUT?	W —WHEREABOUT?
X —X-RAY PROCEDURE	X —X-RAY SHADOW	X —X-RAY SHADOW
Y —YOUR PATIENT DATA	Y —YOUR PATIENT DATA	Y —YOUR PATIENT DATA
Z —ZANY SHADOW	Z —ZANY SHADOW: ARTIFACT, COMPOSITE	Z —ZANY SHADOW

+ Exact numbers, measurements and staging may be coded in parenthesis.
* Denotes functional as distinct from structural changes.
— Denotes a qualifying category.

Figure 31. The major alphabetic coding categories for radiology reports used in the CLIP system.[159] (Reproduced with permission from Simon, M. *et al.* Computerized Radiology Reporting Using Coded Language. *Radiology 113*, 343–349, 1974. Copyright RSNA.)

A similar alphanumeric system, initially called Radiologic Diagnoses Instantly Accessed and Transmitted Electronically (RADIATE) and subsequently renamed Missouri Automated Reporting System (MARS), was developed using IBM mainframe computers and cathode ray terminals.[160,161] Figure 32 shows the list of modifier codes for the RADIATE system.

A—Right	K—Small	U—Healing	4—Single	&—Benign
B—Left	L—Medium	V—Healed	5—Multiple	----Malignant
C—Proximal	M—Large	W—Acute	6—Diffused	*---Metastatic
D—Distal	N—Minimal	X—Subacute	7—Generalized	)---Primary
E—Middle	O—Maximal	Y—Chronic	8—Congenital	,---Secondary
F—Medial	P—Moderate	Z—Worse	9—Acquired	
G—Lateral	Q—Severe	0—Improved		
H—Anterior				
I—Posterior	S—Superior			
J—Bilateral	T—Inferior			

Enter up to 8 modifier codes (@ for no entry, = for free text)

Figure 32. Alphanumeric modifier codes used in the RADIATE system to capture structured reports in 1969.[160] (Reproduced with permission from Templeton, A. W. *et al.* Radiate—Updated and Redesigned for Multiple Cathode-Ray Tube Terminals. *Radiology 92,* 30–36, 1969. Copyright RSNA.)

Researchers at the LDS Hospital in Utah subsequently developed a similar system to capture and report radiologic findings. The system enabled radiologists to check boxes on paper forms, specifying the findings, severity, size, number, time course, and confidence level. Then the radiologist selected one of the diagnoses listed on the request form or dictated a short report.

A medical secretary subsequently entered the check box information into the computer, where it was available for review at hospital nursing stations. This need for clerical support foreshadowed the disadvantages of some structured reporting systems: They can be incompatible with efficient radiology documentation.

Touch Screens

A radiology reporting system developed by Dr. Paul Wheeler has been used routinely at Johns Hopkins Hospital since 1972,[162] a remarkable achievement. The system presents a study-specific touch panel filled with anatomic and pathologic terms. Figure 33 shows the overall computer set-up back in the 1970s, including a close-up of a touch panel to capture report information for a hand radiograph.

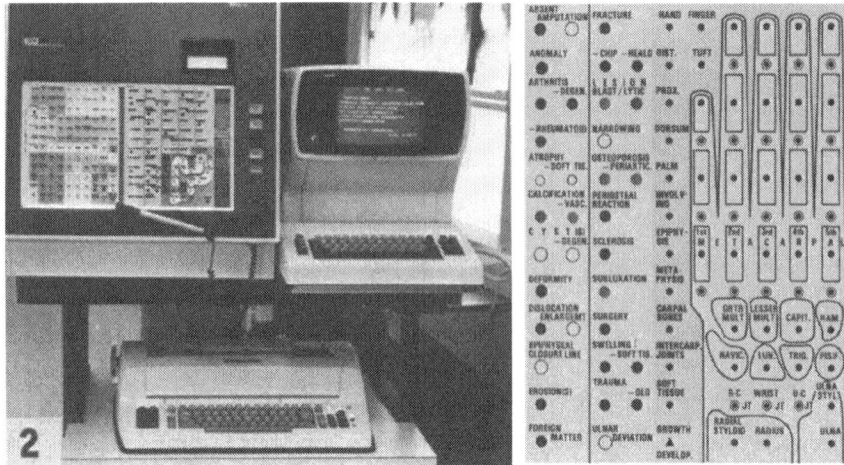

Figure 33. The computer set-up for the Johns Hopkins structured radiology reporting system (left) and an electronic touch panel for hand-wrist-finger radiographs (right).[162] (Reproduced with permission from Wheeler, P. S., Simborg, D. W. & Gitlin, J. N. The Johns Hopkins Radiology Reporting System. *Radiology 119*, 315–319, 1976. Copyright RSNA.)

This system was adapted and updated to run on more modern computer hardware.[163] Each selection causes a text phrase to be added to the report. Users say the system can be quite efficient once the radiologist learns the many phrase options available for each study type.

Mark-Sense Forms

One of the only early attempts to commercialize structured reporting, called RAPORT, was licensed by General Electric Medical Systems from the University of California, San Francisco.[164] At one point in the mid 1970s, it was operational in more than 25 hospital radiology practices of various types and sizes.[165,166] Figure 34 shows the mark-sense forms (similar to those used for the SAT and other standardized tests), which were later optically decoded by a computer mark reader. Information from the forms was combined with the radiologist's dictation, which was transcribed in parallel. Information about the use of the RAPORT system is scarce, but one can only assume it suffered from the same productivity problems as other early structured reporting systems.

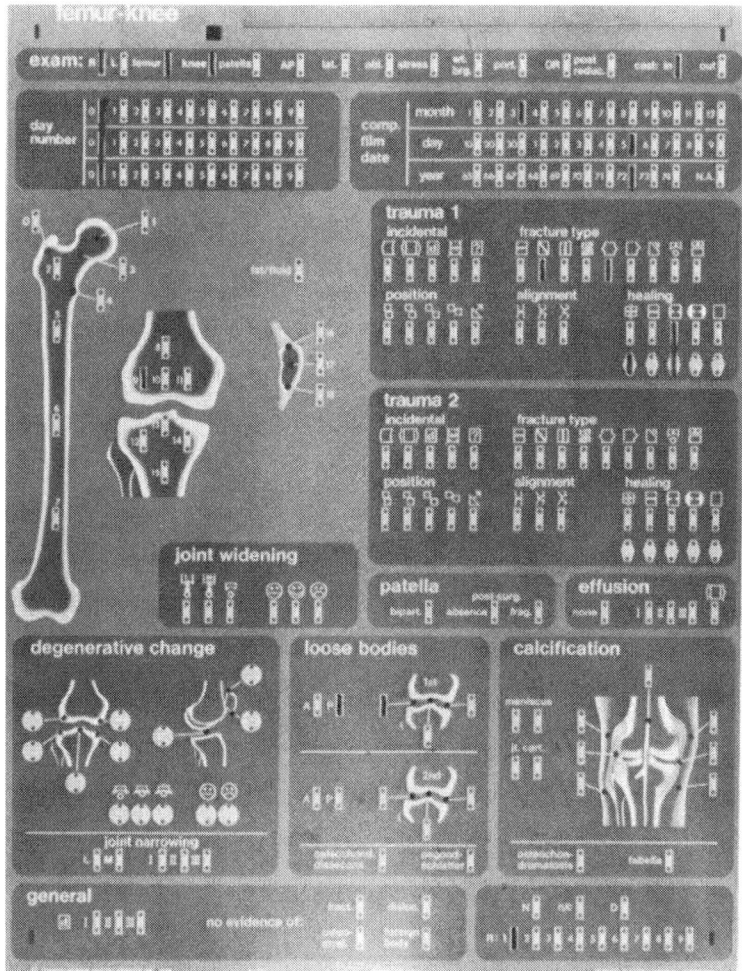

Figure 34. A mark-sense form used by the commercial RAPORT system to capture structured reports in 1973.[164] (Reproduced with permission from Mani, R. L. & Jones, M. D. MSF: A Computer-Assisted Radiologic Reporting System. *Radiology 108,* 587–596, 1973. Copyright RSNA.)

IBM, a major computer manufacturer at the time, also developed a radiology reporting system based on mark-sense forms that were later read by a computer.[167] This system was successfully tested on 26,000 radiographs of healthy workers. Figure 35 shows a portion of one of these forms, intended for radiographic studies of the chest.

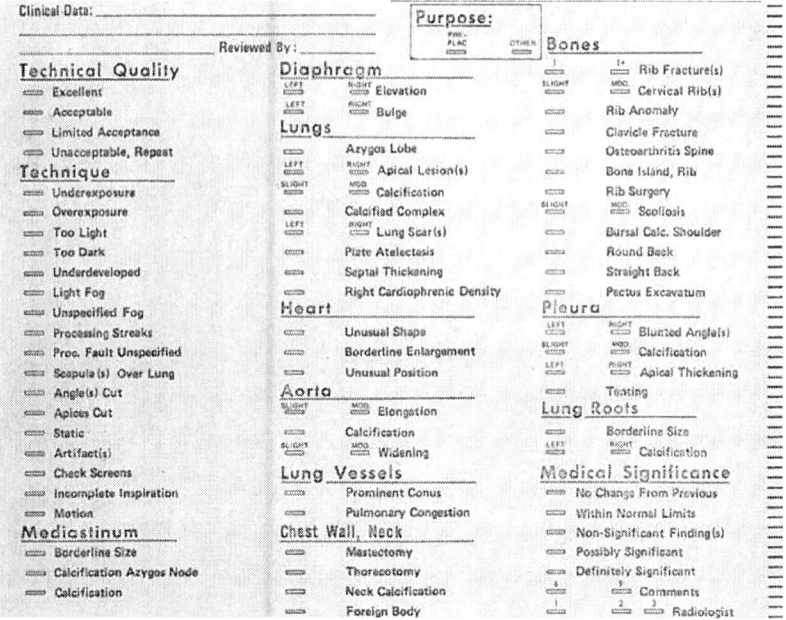

Figure 35. A portion of a mark-sense form developed by IBM to
capture structured reports of chest radiographs.[167]
(Reproduced with permission from Sherman, R. S. An
Automated System for Recording Reports of Chest
Roentgenograms. *Am J Roentgenol 117,* 848–854 (1973).
Copyright ARRS.)

Each choice on the form created a phrase in an automatically generated narrative report. For example, marking the "Unusual Shape" item under "Heart" on the form in Figure 35 resulted in the sentence "The heart shape is a little unusual."

Capturing and generating structured reports was an impressive feat given the computing technology of the 1960s and 1970s. But most of these systems could not be sustained in the clinical environment. Computing power, memory, and storage capacity were insufficient. The keyboard and character-based computer screens were markedly inefficient user interfaces, and the terminology and symbol systems were not standardized or easily learned. As a result, these systems were cumbersome and slow for radiologists to use and were never widely adopted.

Speech Recognition

*Supercomputers will achieve one human brain capacity by 2010,
and personal computers will do so by about 2020.*
—Ray Kurzweil

In the late 1980s, I worked as a graduate student in a computer science laboratory at Stanford University. I distinctly remember an eminent Silicon Valley computer scientist breathlessly describing the speech recognition system he had just seen, demonstrated by its creator, an engineer named Ray Kurzweil: "A user speaks into Kurzweil's system and the computer prints out the words!" Soon thereafter, in 1986, the Kurzweil Applied Intelligence Corporation produced the first automated speech recognition system. After laborious training, the system could correctly recognize about 1,000 words at a rate of 40 words per minute. The system ran on a personal computer with an extra board that provided sound processing capabilities. (Personal computers of those days typically had processor speeds of 5 MHz, 256 Kbytes of RAM, and three card slots for "extra" capabilities such as sound processing and memory expansion.)

Unfortunately, the system achieved an accuracy of only about 85% and required the user to pause between every word.[168] Medical professionals were the initial target market, but sales were glacially slow. Why? Nobody. Dictates. Like. This. The Kurzweil system was unlikely to serve as an efficient replacement for most typical dictation tasks. And few busy physicians would tolerate errors in one to two words out of every 10.

The Kurzweil system was the first of many false starts in the long history of commercial medical speech recognition systems. Yet, the innovations of Ray Kurzweil and other inventors dating back to the late 19th century ultimately led to today's systems. For those interested in the origins of transcription and speech recognition business, the remainder of this chapter reviews the historical factors that shaped today's market.

Alexander Graham Bell and Dictaphone

Before anything else, preparation is the key to success.
—Alexander Graham Bell

The story of automated speech recognition starts with the scientist and inventor, Alexander Graham Bell. In 1886, just 5 years after his Volta Laboratory was first established in the Georgetown area of Washington, DC, Bell patented a device to record the human voice on a wax cylinder and founded the Volta Graphophone Company to manufacture it. The Dictaphone brand was first trademarked several years thereafter, in 1907. A second spin-off of the Bell laboratory was focused on a similar recording process that used discs. After a series of mergers and splits, the disc company became Columbia Records. In 1923, the Dictaphone Company spun out of the music label to focus on the dictation and transcription business. Soon, the descendants of Alexander Graham Bell's early recording systems became products called "Dictaphones" and "phonographs"—familiar names that persisted over the ensuing decades.

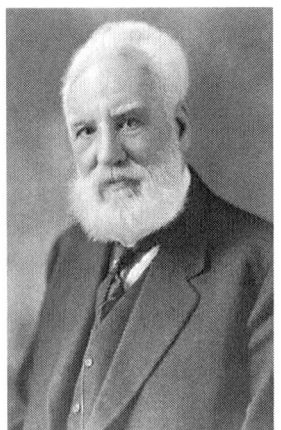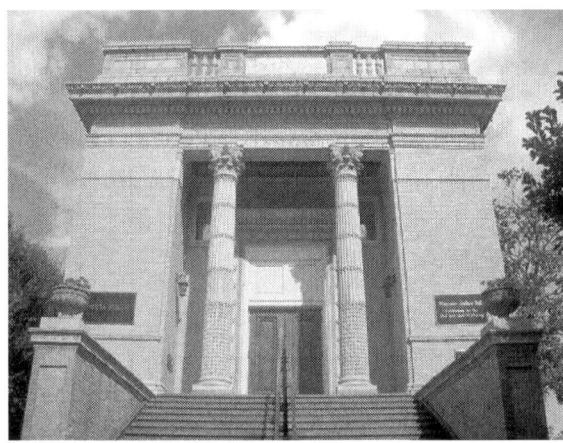

Figure 36. Alexander Graham Bell and his Volta Laboratory, founded in 1881. (Left: Expired copyright. Right: Photograph distributed under a CC BY-SA 3.0 license.)

Bell's first Dictaphone was a disruptive innovation: It replaced human stenographers. As the United States shifted from an agrarian to an industrial economy during the 19th century, the stenography profession emerged to meet the growing need to record speech in real time. An individual stenographer used "shorthand" to create an accurate written record of speech at a conversational pace. (My grandmother, who was born in 1898 and worked as a secretary at Bell Telephone, was quite proud of the speed and accuracy of her shorthand skills.)

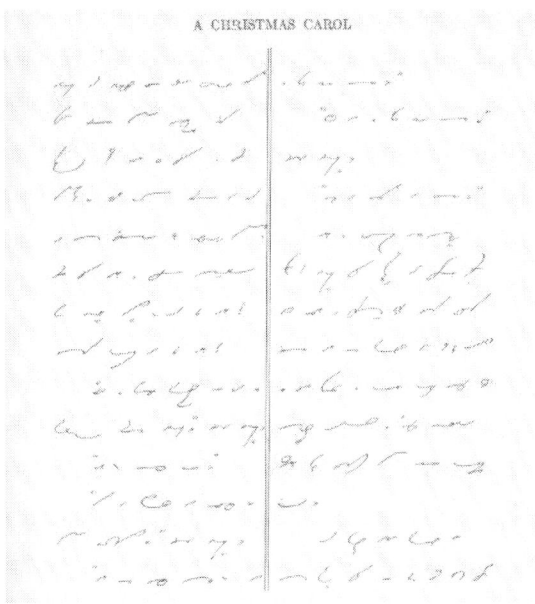

Figure 37. A sample of shorthand stenography, which enabled clerical staff to record speech at a conversational pace. This "Gregg" form of shorthand was the most common in the United States.

Dictaphone and its competitors offered all manner of recording devices, including wax cylinders and belts, to be later transcribed by the "transcription pool." One of the more popular technologies, developed after World War II was "Dictabelt" technology, which cut a mechanical groove in a plastic belt.

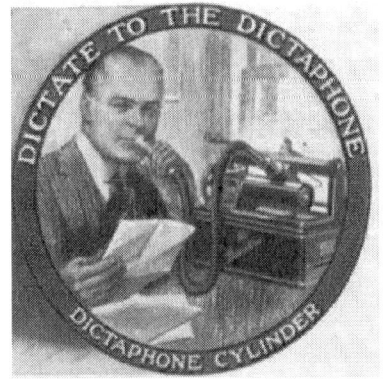
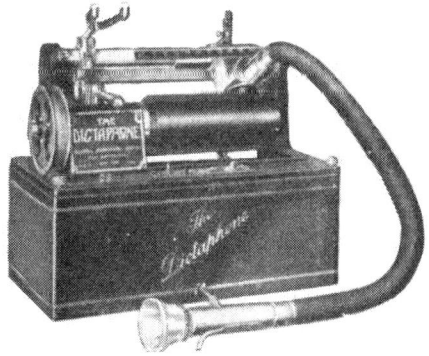

Figure 38. A Dictaphone magazine advertisement from 1917 and a Dictaphone machine similar to the one it featured.

Wax and plastic grooves eventually gave way to modern magnetic recording technologies.[169] In the 1970s, Dictaphone introduced "endless loop" recording on a magnetic tape, branded as a "Thought Tank." I remember hearing older radiologists refer to "tank-based" dictation systems. These systems were particularly popular in medicine because they didn't require the distribution and collection of tapes.

Nevertheless, when portable cassette tapes became inexpensive, many radiology departments replaced their tank systems with cassette tape recorders. A clerk collected full cassette tapes and brought back erased empties. This system was decidedly modern compared with a wax cylinder. But when tapes were lost, or erased by mistake, half a day's dictation work needed to be reproduced, usually by the radiology resident. (I speak from experience.)

As the recording technology and dictation market evolved, Dictaphone Corporation remained a leading provider of solutions to radiologists and other medical professionals. The Lanier Corporation, Dictaphone's only major direct competitor at the time, remained relatively weak until it was sold in 2002.

When phone-based digital recording systems became feasible in the 1980s, many practices outsourced the transcription pool to regional or national transcription companies. As these transcription companies grew to achieve national scope, a new disruptive innovation would spell the end of the radiology transcription market altogether: speech recognition.

The Advent of Automated Speech Recognition

*We wanted to do something that would be practical and useful
and more than a paper on a library shelf.*
–Janet Baker, PhD[170]

Ray Kurzweil was not the only futuristic thinker to see the potential of the automated speech recognition market. In the 1980s, Dr. James Baker, a computer scientist and distinguished professor at Carnegie Mellon University, and his wife Janet Baker, a PhD biophysicist, met in graduate school and yearned to work together on an important problem that leveraged the growing power of computers.[170,171] Automated speech recognition fit the bill. The Bakers used $35,000 of their own money to found Dragon Systems. Its first product, released in 1990 just a few years after Kurzweil's unit, recognized speech one word at a time, just like the Kurzweil system, and was not well received.[172] But the Bakers persevered, and after an infusion of capital from disk drive maker Seagate, they released the first continuous speech recognition product, Dragon Naturally Speaking, to widespread acclaim.

The late 1990s became the heyday of speech recognition, with many experts predicting the extinction of keyboards. Lernout and Hauspie (L&H), a Belgian speech technology colossus, acquired the Kurzweil technology and developed a continuous speech recognition product. During that time, Philips and IBM offered competing continuous speech recognition engines (SpeechMagic and ViaVoice, respectively), which competed against the Dragon and L&H systems. All of these systems promised accuracy in the 95% range, but most observers believed the Dragon speech engine was superior for medical applications. Through extraordinary skill and perseverance, the Bakers' speech technology achieved market dominance, although a fateful decision would deprive them of major financial rewards from their innovative work.

Speech Recognition in the Clinical Environment

Speech recognition will be most successful when it's invisible, just incorporated into things as another way of interacting.
–Janet Baker, PhD[170]

As medical speech recognition software improved, its manufacturers soon recognized a challenging obstacle: It takes more than great speech recognition accuracy to make a system function in a clinical environment. Consumer speech products did not integrate with the clinical systems that stored and distributed radiology reports. Few radiology practices would purchase consumer speech recognition software off the shelf. Most practices demanded better system integration and held on to their wallets.

Several health information technology businesses were formed in response to these imperatives. These new companies built systems that received radiology orders electronically over the network and returned completed reports in the same manner. Talk Technology, one of the early pioneers of this integrated approach, initially licensed the IBM speech recognition engine. Both Philips and L&H developed their own clinical product lines. Articulate Systems, a small start-up, developed radiology reporting software called PowerScribe, based on the Dragon engine. These systems not only exchanged orders and reports, but also solved many other complexities of radiology reporting. They could manage associated exams, when a single report served as the documentation for more than one order (e.g., radiographic study of the hand and wrist dictated together). And they accommodated trainee work flow common in many academic institutions, when resident dic-tations must be reviewed and edited before the final signature of the attend-ing radiologist.

Corporate Consolidation and Scandal

Rather fail with honor than succeed by fraud.
–Sophocles

Several large radiology practices adopted clinical speech recognition sys-tems in the early 2000s, including my own at the University of Pennsylvania. But the Internet bubble at the turn of the millennium was a time of chaotic consolidation for speech recognition vendors. IBM stopped supporting its speech engine, and Talk Technology soon substituted the Dragon engine in its products. L&H went on a buying binge, acquiring the market-leading Dragon Systems, as well as Articulate Systems, and the staid Dictaphone Cor-poration, which had no significant speech technology but had a long list of transcription clients who were also potential speech recognition customers.

Unfortunately, L&H went bankrupt in 2001 due to a high profile account-ing scandal, leaving the Bakers empty handed. (Both Lernout and Hauspie received a jail sentence.) Dictaphone was spun off as a private company, for the first time with its own speech recognition technology: the PowerScribe product line. The remaining speech recognition assets of L&H, including the valuable Dragon engine, were sold to ScanSoft, a document scanning com-pany founded by Ray Kurzweil. Talk Technology was acquired by Agfa in 2001.

The Current Market Landscape

Competition is not only the basis of protection to the consumer,
but is the incentive to progress.
–Herbert Hoover[173]

Since the bankruptcy of L&H, the speech recognition market has under-gone substantial additional consolidation, led by ScanSoft. In 2005, ScanSoft purchased Nuance, a spin-off from SRI International that had developed speech recognition technology for call centers and secret government pro-jects. The new company assumed the Nuance name and acquired most of the remaining speech recognition companies, including Dictaphone and its PowerScribe product in 2006, radiology speech start-up Commissure in 2007, Philips U.S. speech business in 2008, IBM's speech patent portfolio in 2009, and Apple-centric MacSpeech in 2010. More recently, Nuance has focused its acquisitions on voice-enabling technologies, including the wizardry behind

Siri, the speech recognition application in Apple's mobile devices.[174] As this consolidation occurred, the incremental adoption of speech recognition has grown steadily, increasing from about 5% of radiology practices in the late 1990s, to the vast majority today.

The strong return on investment drove much of this growth: Speech recognition systems typically pay for themselves in reduced transcription costs over about a year. Thus, they generate significant savings over time: In some cases, more than $25,000 annually per radiologist. But many radiologists resisted adopting this new technology because of its effect on radiologist productivity and work flow. Academic radiology departments were the earliest adopters, probably because their management structure is hierarchical rather than consensus- or committee-based, reducing the influence of resisters. Some practices included report turnaround time and speech recognition usage in their financial incentive plans to ensure the new systems were adopted by radiologists, despite objections.

Nuance Communications is currently the market share leader in medical speech recognition technology. The strongest competitor to Nuance is likely M*Modal, which got its start much like Nuance, by using technologies originally developed for the intelligence community. Rather than using the purely syntactic analysis of the Dragon engine, the M*Modal engine uses semantics, natural language processing, and contextual information to enhance recognition. The same technologies extract key concepts from radiology reports for use in automated coding and other applications. In 2010, M*Modal was acquired by MedQuist, one of the largest medical transcription outsourcers, who retained the M*Modal brand. Several other reporting vendors, including DR Systems (recently acquired by Merge, which was then acquired by IBM), Carestream, and Epic serve smaller radiology market segments.

Both Nuance and M*Modal represent powerhouse partnerships between old-school transcription companies (Dictaphone and MedQuist, respectively) and high-technology speech recognition developers (Dragon and M*Modal, respectively). It will be interesting to watch these vendors compete and evolve in the radiology reporting market.

Chapter 8:
Toward Structured Reporting

I often say that when you can measure what you are speaking about, and express it in numbers, you know something about it; but when you cannot measure it, when you cannot express it in numbers, your knowledge is of a meagre and unsatisfactory kind.
—*Sir William Thomson (Lord Kelvin)*

(Note: Portions of this chapter were adapted with permission from references [175–179].)

Dr. Preston Hickey was one of the foremost advocates for radiology professionalism in the early 20th century and a giant in the new discipline of radiology. His love for photography led him to purchase one of the first x-ray machines in Michigan, ultimately leading to his appointment as chair of the radiology department at the University of Michigan. As one of the founding members of what later became the American Roentgen Ray Society, Dr. Hickey helped instill professional discipline into the group and edited its journal during its earliest years. He first coined the term *radiograph* and was the first to use the term *interpretation* to describe the contents of the report. He went on to pioneer the oblique radiograph and the use of compression to reduce scatter.[23]

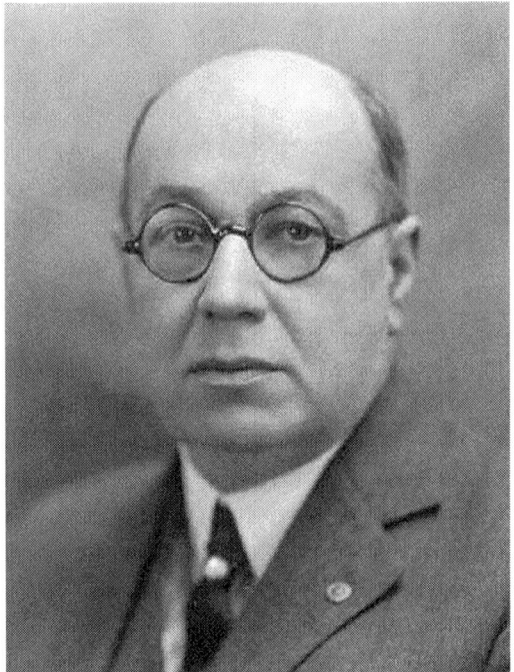

Figure 39. Preston Hickey, a pioneer in the use of standard language in radiology reports. (Reproduced with permission from the Clendening Library Portrait Collection, University of Kansas.)

Dr. Hickey also distinguished himself as an early advocate for improved radiology reporting. Hickey's landmark work was prompted by his attendance at a surgical congress dedicated to the diagnosis and prognosis of bone sarcomas, where several radiology reports from prestigious hospitals were read. He concluded "from these reports, it was difficult to determine, in the majority of cases, the actual bone condition encountered," and he noted that the surgeons in the audience naturally concluded that radiography could contribute very little value to the epidemiology of sarcomas.

To address these problems, Hickey recommended a standard language and format for radiology reports:

Reports filed in hospitals should be scientifically accurate and should follow an accepted nomenclature, so as to have value in a statistical sense.

Hickey also advocated that reports be "written in a manner ... that would convey distinct ideas as to the conditions present." (Today, this recommendation sounds so obvious as to be laughable.)

As a result of his investigations, Dr. Hickey advocated that "an attempt should be made to standardize roentgen ray reports," including use of "a standardized nomenclature." As an example, he proposed the standard fracture report from Dr. Harold J. Pierce, shown in Figure 40.

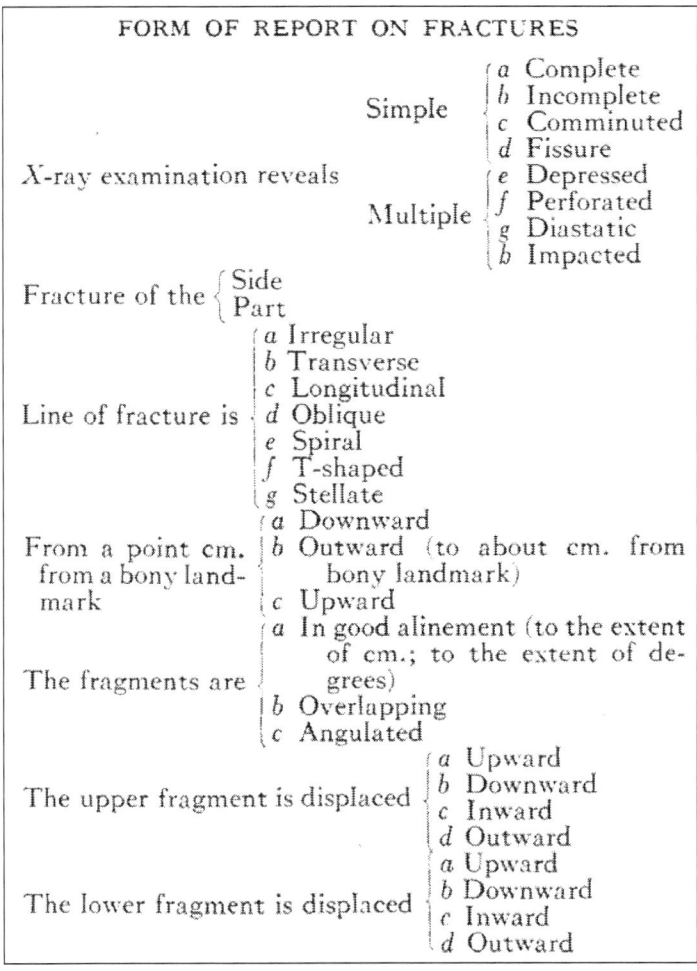

Figure 40. A standard form used by Dr. Harold Pierce to record radiology findings for images showing fractures.[5]

Radiologists today would call Hickey's sensible proposal for standardized reports "structured reporting."

Radiology Reporting a Century Later

The mouse produces two analog voltages ... in proportion to the X or Y movement over the table top. These voltages control the coordinates of a tracking spot with which the user may "point" to positions on the screen.
—*Douglas C. Engelbart and William K. English*[180]

Despite Dr. Hickey's exhortations, why have radiology reporting processes remained essentially unchanged for almost 100 years? Primarily because they optimize the efficiency of the radiologist. It is relatively easy for a radiologist to pick up a microphone and create a free-form narrative that describes aspects of the image as they come to mind. Likewise, it is easy for those reports to be transcribed and presented to the radiologist, who quickly skims and signs them.

But the arrival in the 1990s of high-resolution monitors driven by a computer mouse led many to believe that radiology reporting systems modeled after Dr. Hickey's approach were feasible.[181,182] Users gave favorable reviews to the UltraSTAR system, an experimental ultrasound structured reporting system based on early Apple computers.[183] Newly available Internet technologies also showed appeal and promise for structured reporting.[184] The benefits of structured data capture were also becoming clear in other medical specialties, including pediatrics,[185] emergency medicine,[186] obstetrics,[187] mental health,[188] and gastrointestinal endoscopy.[189]

The 1994 Mammography Quality Standards Act (MQSA), which required reporting and tracking of certain elements of the radiology report, became another strong driver of change. Major RIS vendors responded by incorporating breast image reporting systems into their products. A number of independent vendors successfully marketed systems for mammography reporting, including PenRad (Buffalo, MN), MRS (Lynwood, WA), and MagView (Burtonsville, MD). Ultrasound and cardiology vendors incorporated structured reporting features into their imaging systems. A new DICOM structured reporting (DICOM-SR) standard was approved in 2000.[190]

Venture capitalists and other investors soon perceived structured reporting as an area ripe for investment. Several young companies, including eDictation,[191] StructuRad,[192] and PointDx, began to develop products for the full spectrum of radiology studies, not just breast imaging or ultrasound. Hope filled the air.

But today, even a casual observer will note that none of these businesses succeeded. We have not yet arrived at a world of widespread adoption of structured reporting. eDictation ceased operations in 2004. PointDx was purchased by a RIS company that never brought its structured reporting product to market. StructuRad also apparently has closed its doors.

Structured Reporting: A Case Study

Why did this generation of reporting systems fail to take hold? I am uniquely qualified to answer that question because I founded eDictation, wrote the first version of the software, and subsequently served as its chief executive officer. Those experiences gave me an acute sense of the miscalculations of its early advocates. For example, the company's original business plan called for essentially all of the radiology report to be captured by using point-and-click, in part because speech recognition at the time was in its early days and was experiencing a serious backlash among radiologists.

Although there was much speculation at the time about the effect of structured reporting systems on the quality of radiology reports, almost no data had been produced to support these assessments. Some proponents, including me, erroneously believed that creating structured reports could be faster than conventional reporting methods.

The eDictation system was typical for its day and serves as a representative case study of that era's structured radiology reporting systems. The reports created by the system were organized in sections with headings, contained a consistent ordering of observations, and used terms drawn from a lexicon. The system emphasized the selection of standard reporting elements from an electronic menu,[193] while allowing additional narrative to be dictated by using speech recognition. (When a radiologist selected the "Text" tab in Figure 41, the Dragon Naturally Speaking speech engine was invoked.)

To create a structured sentence in the eDictation system, the user first selected an anatomic structure from an anatomic hierarchy tailored to the study being reported. When an anatomic structure was selected, a menu of observations appeared, specific to the chosen anatomy, as shown in Figure 41. eDictation then created a narrative sentence corresponding to the anatomy and finding chosen: "A synovial effusion is present in the knee joint."

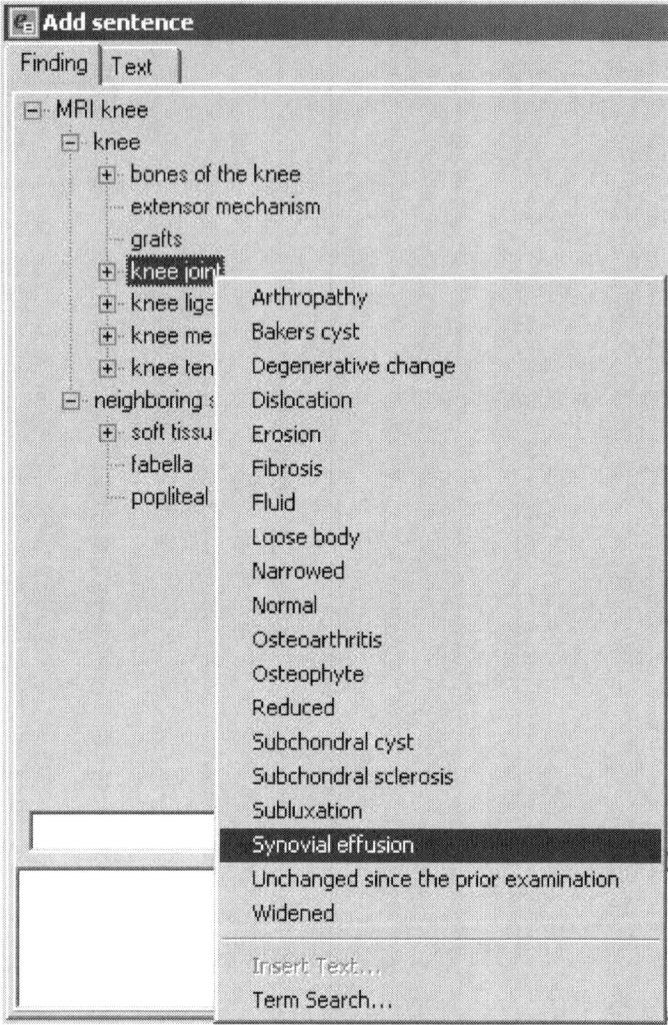

Figure 41. The eDictation method of creating report sentences. Based on the selected anatomy, a tailored menu of findings appeared. The system automatically generated a sentence corresponding to the selections, in this case, "A synovial effusion is present in the knee joint."

Users could modify existing sentences with structured modifiers. Figure 42 shows a "Small" modifier being applied.

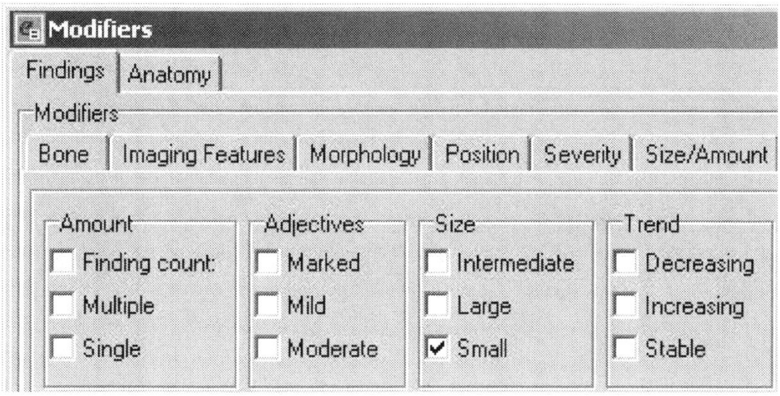

Figure 42. eDictation's modifier interface. Several types of modifiers were available.

Users could also specify one of seven confidences levels, from "Definitely" to "Definitely Not," with "Maybe," "Probably," and "Unsure" in between. After each selection, the corresponding sentence was modified accordingly. In this case, the final sentence is "A small synovial effusion probably is present in the knee joint."

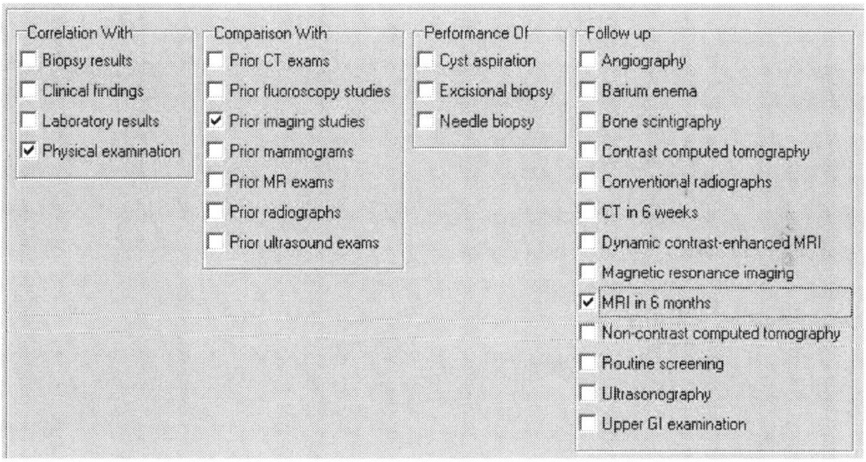

Figure 43. An example of eDictation's user interface for recommendations, which were included in a separate section of the report. The checked boxes indicate the recommendations that the radiologist would like to include in the report.

eDictation also enabled its users to select from a wide range of structured recommendations. Figure 43 shows three selected recommendations the user wishes to include in the report.

The user could decide which findings from the body of the report were crucial enough to highlight in the Impression section.

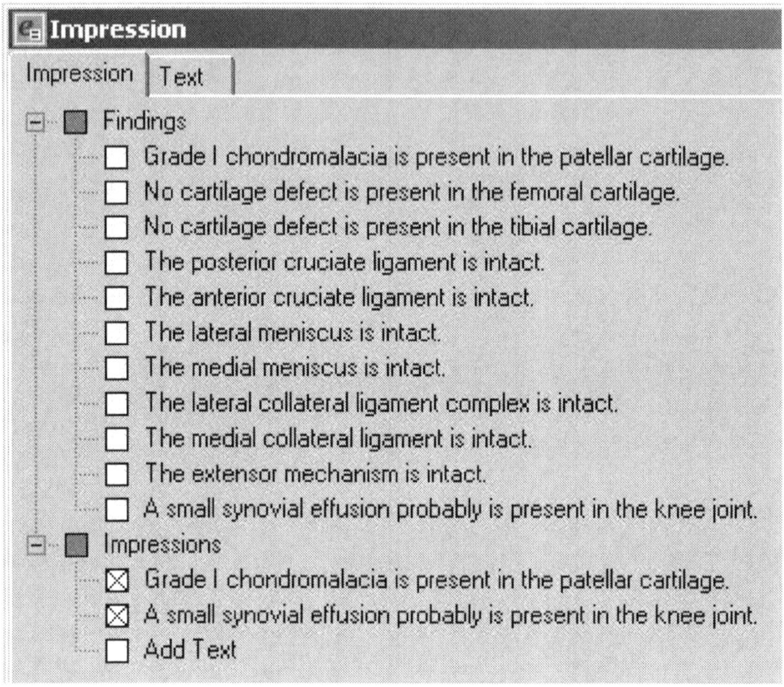

Figure 44. eDictation's Impression selection interface. The user decided which sentences from the report were sufficiently important to include in the Impression section.

Once the radiologist was satisfied with the narrative report displayed by the system, the report could be reviewed and signed. As shown in Figure 45, the final form of the report was very similar to most other radiology reports.

Referring Physician3741, MD
973 Tabitha Road
Haslip, NJ 08010

Patient Name: Oliver Twist
MRN: 9384575
DOB: 11 / 05 / 1967

Examination: MRI knee (Left)

Technique:
Axial T1-weighted MR images, T1-weighted sagittal MR images, coronal T1-weighted MR images, axial T2-weighted MR images, T2-weighted sagittal MR images, and coronal T2-weighted MR images were obtained.

Findings:
Grade I chondromalacia is present in the patellar cartilage. No cartilage defect is present in the femoral cartilage. No cartilage defect is present in the tibial cartilage. The posterior cruciate ligament is intact. The anterior cruciate ligament is intact. The lateral meniscus is intact. The medial meniscus is intact. The lateral collateral ligament complex is intact. The medial collateral ligament is intact. The extensor mechanism is intact. A small synovial effusion probably is present in the knee joint.

Correlation with physical examination, comparison with prior imaging studies, and follow up MRI in 6 months is recommended.

Impression:

1. **Grade I chondromalacia is present in the patellar cartilage.**
2. **A small synovial effusion probably is present in the knee joint.**

Figure 45. The final form of an eDictation report, which was compatible with reports produced using conventional dictation.

But eDictation reports had a crucial difference. By creating the report through structured entry, the user had simultaneously created an underlying database of discrete information.

Through the lens of today's technology, there is much to critique about the eDictation interface: Many of its shortcomings were due to the technologic limitations of the time. Reliable development environments for web software were not yet available, and a comprehensive standard lexicon to represent the information in a radiology report did not yet exist.[194]

The developers of eDictation (myself included) began with a flawed premise: Radiologists despised speech recognition (correct) and would therefore never adopt it (incorrect). They assumed that radiologists would enter the vast majority of report information through point-and-click. As a result, the system contained too many windows, tabs, check boxes, and clicks. Although eDictation allowed dictation of narrative text, doing so itself required a click.

And of course, many present-day users would be repelled by the gray background, clunky icons, and unglamorous fonts. But those were the graphic elements available in the best software tools of the day.

A Rigorous Evaluation

I take pride in the fact that eDictation was rigorously evaluated—prospectively compared with conventional dictation in an experiment designed to show the effect of structured reporting on the accuracy and completeness of radiology reports.[195] Twenty-five brain MR imaging studies were reviewed in two distinct phases by two separate groups of residents: one using eDictation and the other using conventional dictation.

The study results were surprising, at least to advocates of structured reporting. The use of the structured reporting system caused a clinically significant *decrease* in the completeness and accuracy of radiology reports. An accompanying survey revealed that users found the system overly constraining and inefficient to use. Paradoxically, despite these complaints, the vast majority of respondents believed that structured reporting was a good idea.

When a high-quality clinical trial yields surprising answers, it is revealing to analyze the preconceptions that led us to imagine the opposite result. One answer can be found by examining the successes of structured reporting systems to date: These systems are most widely adopted in breast imaging,[196] cardiology,[197,198] and gastroenterology[199]— disciplines that survey a limited anatomic area to detect a restricted set of diseases. In that setting, manageable template sets can be developed.

Case mix may also play a role. A large proportion of the exams performed by breast imagers, cardiologists, and gastroenterologists are normal or screening studies, which often can be reported in a single click by invoking a template.

Lessons Learned

The eDictation experience provides a clear view of an early wrong turn on the road to structured reporting systems. Looking back, the mistakes seem obvious. Like other rational fee-for-service workers, radiologists will resist adopting a system that slows them down. The tangible benefits of the underlying structured data, such as registry reporting, automated recommendation follow-up, and real-time decision support, are only now being realized. Regulatory and financial incentives, which are strong drivers of the adoption of new systems, were absent outside breast imaging a decade ago, but are becoming stronger every year. And the seamless integration of speech recognition and voice commands into an efficient user interface has finally become a reality.

As the regulatory imperatives of structured reporting become impossible to resist, and the technologic developments take hold, we can expect an increasing variety of novel structured reporting products to enable the efficient creation of both simple and complex reports.[179,200]

Structured Reporting: A Definition

The term *structured reporting* has become confusing to some, because it is employed to describe such a disparate collection of reporting techniques. Some experts argue that radiology reports are already structured, albeit in a rather loose and imperfect manner, because they follow a format that includes consistent section headings. To others, the term embodies new techniques, supported by referring clinicians, who prefer itemized reports with separate headings for every organ system in a consistent order.[24,40–42] Purists use structured reporting as a synonym for automated reporting software systems such as eDictation, which substitute point-and-click data capture for dictation. (Pathologists call this "synoptic reporting.")

Rather than attempt to adjudicate these differences, we will evaluate structured reporting as simply another way to improve the radiology report so it can better serve its purpose: communication. Structured reports make radiology information easily accessible and reusable in an era of EMRs. So our discussion of structured reporting as a means to improve radiology reporting will focus on three distinct attributes of the report: *format*, *organization*, and *terminology*.

Uniform Logical Format

All high-quality reports, including structured reports, should follow a uniform format. The *format* of any document refers to the actual layout of the content as seen by the reader. A visually appealing and logical format is central to customer satisfaction and to the efficient and accurate transfer of information. We know a great deal about how to format information for optimal communication and rapid information retrieval, but this science has only rarely been applied to the formatting and display of radiology reports.

Tip: Review the format of your reports as they appear to referring clinicians. Report formats often are garbled as they pass through the primitive interfaces that connect systems today. A few simple and obvious changes might give your reports a more professional appearance and significantly improve referring clinicians' perception of your practice.

Consistent Organization

When we look up an address, we find the information in a consistent order: street number, street name, city, state, and zip code. Standard ordering makes it easy for the reader to process and understand information. Our clinical colleagues deserve no less from radiology reports.

For a given examination and clinical context, structured reports should list the same major elements in the same order, regardless of the author. Most practices already routinely divide the report into sections with headings. (In Chapter 6 we proposed standard section headings and the information each section should include.) Likewise, subspecialty imaging divisions should agree on an appropriate order for imaging observations according to anatomic or physiologic functional units, with observations listed under each one. Use of reporting templates can encourage consistent and organized reports.

Although some purists discount the power of simply standardizing the format and organization of radiology reports, simple report structure has great potential to improve patient outcomes, even when radiologists have no restrictions on the text that can be placed under each heading. Consistent report organization may be just as important to the satisfaction of referring clinicians as any other aspect of the report.[24,40]

Standard Terminology

Once a practice has agreed on an overall format and organization for their radiology reports, an important question arises: Can we agree on the terminology that should be used to describe normal and abnormal observations? For example, how should the kidney be described on renal ultrasound studies? Are there certain aspects of a liver tumor that should always be mentioned? Do the ICU clinicians who read our portable chest radiograph reports actually prefer that we mention the position of the tip of each tube and catheter in every report?

The notion of *standard terminology* refers to the extent to which the language in a radiology report is agreed upon by the report creator and the report reader. In theory, medical training produces physicians who share a conceptual model of human pathophysiology and use mutually understood language. Ideally, this training prepares physicians to communicate effectively, both orally and by creating and reading narrative text documents. But we do not live in that ideal world; the problems of miscommunication are well documented. A single radiologist reporting two examinations with similar findings can employ very different words and phrases for each of the studies.[201] (See Chapter 9 for an in-depth discussion of terminology for the radiology report.)

A Surprising Consensus Emerges

Although the disruptive changes of eDictation and other upstart structured reporting systems failed to take hold a decade ago, the forces driving change remained in place: the reporting requirements of new payment systems and other regulatory changes, the transformation of radiology practice by information technology, and the growing belief among almost all referring clinicians and many radiologists that standardization of reports is desirable.[24,42] In response to these forces, a gradual transition has begun from fully narrative reports to reports that contain some structured elements.

Most reporting systems lack the features needed to support this transition—a "chicken and egg" problem. Major radiology reporting vendors have not incorporated advanced reporting capabilities into their products because radiologists have not created sophisticated templates that require those capabilities. And radiologists have not created sophisticated templates because the tools radiologists need to create and use advanced templates are not offered by the vendors. The resulting conundrum: Radiologists cannot implement innovative reporting methods because the technology doesn't exist, and the technology doesn't exist because most radiologists weren't asking for it. It took a consensus conference and a national initiative to break the cycle.

The ACR Intersociety Conference

Each summer, the American College of Radiology (ACR) convenes the leadership of dozens of radiology subspecialty organizations to discuss a timely topic of high interest to radiologists. In 2007, the topic of this Intersociety Conference was the radiology report. For several years, I had been advocating that radiologists adopt structured reporting (without much success), so I was asked to lead a breakout group on the topic.

I had low expectations that this group would rally around the notion that radiologists should change their reporting methods. But to my surprise, the leadership of a diverse group of radiology organizations reached consensus on the following key points.[202]

1. Structured reporting is the optimal reporting method, provided that structured reporting tools do not impede radiologist productivity.
2. Reporting tools should enable a hybrid of speech recognition and structured reporting.
3. Radiology professional organizations should create a repository of exemplary reports based on standard vocabulary.

A European focus group later drew similar conclusions.[108]

You may have noticed the "spoonful of sugar" in these recommendations that probably helped the medicine go down: "Do not impede radiologist productivity." Much of the resistance to structured reporting arises out of justifiable apprehension that it will take longer to create a structured report. The second point accommodates this concern by ensuring that speech recognition remains available to radiologists. The third point acknowledges the need for help in creating structured reporting templates. To avoid duplicate effort, professional organizations were asked to develop a resource that all practices could draw upon as they include more structured elements in their reports.

The RSNA Template Library

Largely in response to the consensus formed at that meeting, the Radiological Society of North America (RSNA) created a reporting initiative, which aims to help radiologists create better reports by promoting adoption of clear and consistent templates containing reusable data.[109,203] I chaired this initiative during its early years, convening groups of experts and subspecialty professional societies to create a library of templates for many common imaging exams. The resulting templates are based on standard terminology, developed in collaboration with professional organizations and standards bodies, and are intended to be adapted by radiology practices to accommodate local practice patterns.

The RSNA template library (freely available at www.radreport.org) contains hundreds of templates (in several languages) for common radiology study types; the RSNA templates have been viewed or downloaded millions of times.[204] Expert consensus groups developed these templates to showcase the most detailed structure for every aspect of the report, so these reports probably are not practical to adopt in their entirety. But they can serve as a starting point for practices wishing to standardize their reporting. RSNA recently established an open template library to which any member can contribute (open.radreport.org). This library will provide additional material for radiologists seeking practical templates.

But the users of structured templates still face a serious problem. Our current system of templates operates as though it were designed by a lunatic: A radiologist cannot immediately use the RSNA templates in a vendor-supplied reporting system. Every speech recognition system offers a different template authoring tool. These tools offer little appeal to users and are incompatible with the RSNA library. Therefore, each practice, and sometimes each radiologist, must create a separate set of templates by hand and cannot take advantage of expert knowledge or the work of thousands of other radiologists who have created similar templates. Each vendor stores templates in a different proprietary format, which makes it difficult or impossible to convert those templates to a new reporting system.

Raising the Bar for Radiology Report Templates

Spurred on by user complaints about this byzantine system, reporting vendors soon began working together to create a standard for the exchange of radiology report templates and to define a "floor" for their format and functionality. I and others began working with the vendors under the auspices of Integrating the Healthcare Enterprise (IHE), a standards body, to create a new profile for template exchange called Management of Radiology Report Templates (MRRT).[205]

Our first step was to describe the minimum capabilities of radiology templates. We designed not just fields filled with text, which most reporting systems support today, but also fields containing numbers, dates, and times. Fields can behave like menus, from which predefined choices can be selected. Choices from these menus can be invoked by speech triggers and can themselves invoke other templates, facilitating a speech-driven reporting method that deemphasizes the use of the mouse and the keyboard. New fields can accept data from other sources, such as measurements from the modality and radiation dose information. Because the new template format is based on HTML5,[206] a language used for representing web pages, the new templates offer all basic text formatting capabilities, including boldface, italics, and table formatting. And the text, or any other element of the template, can be annotated with standard terminology.

This new standard creates a method for template exchange that not only enables rapid download of templates from a library into your reporting software, but also enables you to bring your templates with you when you move between radiology practices or change speech recognition vendors. As vendors adopt this new standard, you will soon be able to "go shopping" in the RSNA template library (or a library supplied by your vendor or your practice) from your radiology reading room. After selecting the templates you need, you can download them to your reporting system, edit them there if necessary, and begin using them right away. MRRT does for templates what DICOM does for images.

Radiology Report Search and Analytics

Big data is the world's natural resource for the next century.
—Ginni Rometty

Hearing of all the work required to standardize reports, radiologists retort: Aren't we already able to instantaneously search trillions of Internet web pages by using Google or Bing? Radiology report databases contain at most tens of millions of reports. Why not allow radiologists to dictate as before, then use a Google-like search engine to extract the key information from the narrative report once it is complete?[207]

In fact, related technology is already commercially available from many vendors, who recognize that radiology departments have databases filled with millions of radiology reports, each of which is read once (we hope) but rarely used again. Modern radiology practices are like Sudan and other nations who sit on vast oil reserves but remain poor because they are unable to extract and refine their underground petroleum. These radiology departments are awash in reports but can extract precious little information from them.

Radiology analytics is the refinery that converts the inert riches of radiology report databases into actionable information. Analytics typically begin with text search because radiology data consist primarily of narrative text.

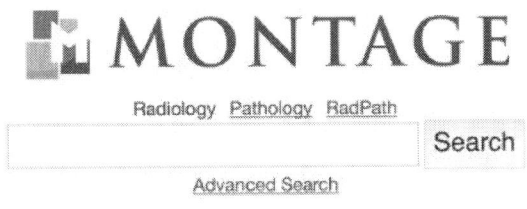

Figure 46. The search screen for Montage Search and Analytics, which is reminiscent of Google. (Reproduced with permission from Montage Healthcare.)

Figure 46 shows the search screen from Montage Search and Analytics, one such analytic tool. (Disclosure: I am a founder, shareholder, and board member of Montage Healthcare.) The search results are typically displayed in a manner familiar to users of search engines. But unlike Google or Bing, radiology search engines provide radiology-specific tools to filter results by modality, to correlate radiology and pathology findings, and to show results on a patient timeline. Figure 47 shows the first two results of a search for "pneumonia."

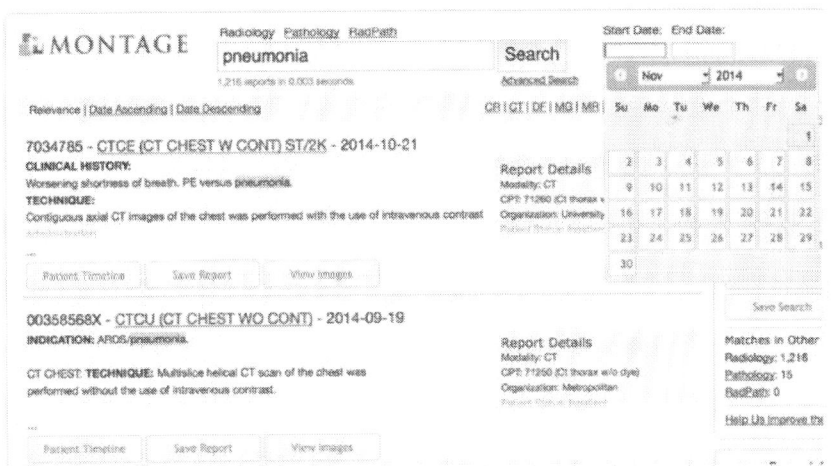

Figure 47. The first two results of a search for pneumonia in a radiology report search tool. These tools enable filtering relevant to radiology, such as by modality. (Reproduced with permission from Montage Healthcare.)

Some radiology search tools can apply standard analytic techniques to the results of a Google-like search. Figure 48 shows an analysis of search results by gender, age, and patient location.

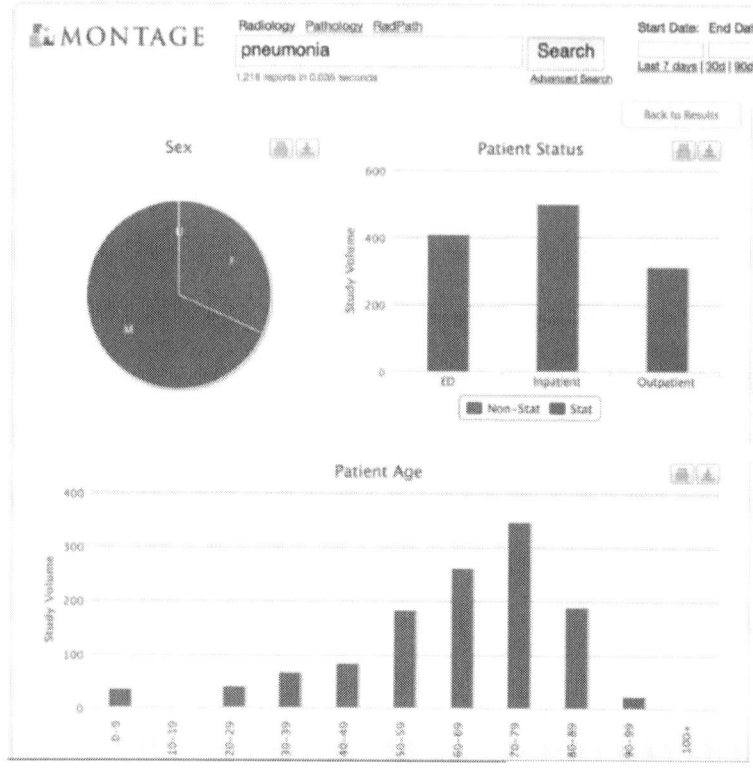

Figure 48. Simple analytics applied to text search results. (Reproduced with permission from Montage Healthcare.)

Of course, these tools also provide more advanced business analytics, such as report turnaround time and analysis of relative value unit (RVU) productivity (see Figure 49).

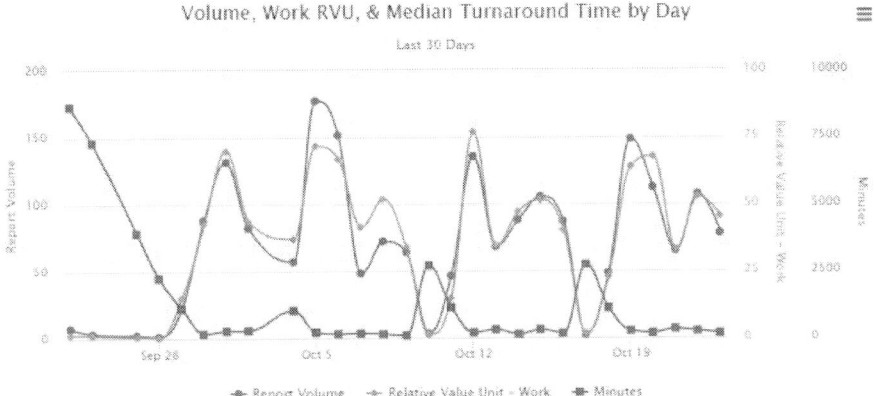

Figure 49. Radiology analytic tools are based not only on text search but also on conventional metrics such as RVU productivity and report signature turnaround time. (Reproduced with permission from Montage Healthcare.)

Finally, some of these analytic tools can perform sophisticated natural language processing to detect specific attributes of a radiology report, such as the critical result dashboard shown in Figure 50. These software systems put the power of large radiology report databases in the hands of practice leaders with no technical analysts as middle men. Whether or not a practice has adopted structured reporting, these systems can provide a powerful business advantage.

Google Has Its Limits

While radiology search engines and the related analytic tools can transform a radiology practice, keep in mind their limitations for searching clinical reports. The most significant limitations relate to negation, uncertainty, and hierarchies—extremely common features of radiology reports but relatively rare on the Internet. For example, if we searched a radiology database for a common pathologic phrase, such as "free air," the vast majority of retrieved reports would contain that phrase as a pertinent negative, such as "There is no evidence of free air." Automated tools are available to detect negated phrases during a report search. The most accurate negation detector has a published sensitivity of 82% and specificity of 96%[208,209]—quite accurate, but still imperfect. For that reason, radiology report search results will never be quite as accurate as Google's.

Synonyms are a second headache for radiology report search algorithms. Synonyms abound in clinical narrative, a characteristic that frustrates conventional text search systems. Consider all the ways in which radiologists express "free air," including all the variations of "intraperitoneal air," "free gas," "intraperitoneal gas," etc. The best search tools automatically expand queries to include not only the entered terms but also their synonyms.

Hierarchical relationships that humans use freely also frustrate text search systems. For example, a search for reports containing the phrase "lung cancer" would not find reports containing the phrase "adenocarcinoma in the lingula" because the words "lung" and "cancer" do not appear. Increasingly, report search systems employ *ontologies* (which is a fancy word for a network of concepts electronically linked together) to enable search systems to expand a query to what the user actually "meant," including hierarchical relationships. But ontologies also have their limitations.

Negation, synonyms, and hierarchies: three reasons there is no free lunch for radiologists who wish to dictate free-text narrative and have the computer figure it out later—which leads us back to structured reporting.

Structured Reporting: A Critical Analysis

The decision to adopt structured reporting is a serious one; the strengths and weaknesses should be considered carefully.[179,210] I am an advocate of structured reporting, and make my case by discussing its salient features below.

The Checklist Analogy

The last time you flew on a commercial airliner, the pilot used a pre-flight checklist to ensure the rudder, flaps, and other plane surfaces were properly configured for takeoff. Pilots use these devices because they reduce the risk of human error, minimize variability, and improve efficiency in the cockpit. How would you feel if the pilot decided not to use a checklist because flying is an "art" and checklists slow him down? Structured reporting plays a role similar to the pilot's checklist. It reduces error, minimizes variability, and counteracts many human failings.

Expert pilots sometimes worry that checklists and autopilots distract them from actually flying the plane, just as radiologists worry that structured reporting tools distract attention from the images themselves. Extending the aviation analogy, the pilot may be so busy with the checklist that he forgets to look out the window and inadvertently flies into the side of a mountain.

But pilots carefully consider when and how they use checklists and other automated aids (and there are ongoing broad efforts to reduce pilots' overuse of autopilot technologies).[211] Radiologists must also remain conscious of when and how often they pay attention to the reporting screen rather than the images, just as they manage other interruptions, such as phone calls and impromptu consultations. In the end, it is the radiologist's responsibility to ensure that enough time has been spent examining the images, just as it is the pilot's responsibility to fly the plane, regardless of checklists or other distractions.

Effects on Training and Education

Do you remember how to do long division? Perhaps just barely. I'll bet 100 years ago, someone with an equivalent education was much better at long division than you are today. They had plenty of practice, because they needed to calculate manually. Electronic calculators are now present on our computers, on our phones, and in the cloud. We can count on their omnipresence to do our division accurately every time. But they have degraded our long division skills. With the advent of global positioning systems (GPS) and turn-by-turn directions, our society's map-reading skills decay every year. And I don't know anyone who can hitch a horse to a buggy. We accept these tradeoffs as signs of progress.

Our level of comfort with the loss of ancient skills probably tracks closely with our feelings about using standard report templates, which remind us to look at each organ in the abdomen. Radiology trainees today are probably less capable of starting with a blank page and producing a cogent dictation than at any time in history. Yet, reports generated by trainees who use templates effectively are probably more consistent and complete than ever before.

How will modern automated reporting systems affect the development of young radiologists? I hope we will see more well-designed experiments to investigate these intriguing questions. The answers will help us optimize radiology training but are unlikely to provide any red flags that deter our progress toward more modern forms of reporting.

Radiologist Decision Support

Any concerns about how structured reporting might degrade the skills of radiologists must be counterbalanced by the benefits. We would all welcome a reporting system that provided relevant clinical information right when we needed it. For a reporting system to know what is relevant to me at a given time, it must understand the current content and structure of my report.

Structured reports are more easily processed by the computer, enabling it to become an intelligent assistant. This intelligent agent could provide the differential diagnosis I need, triggered by the feature I just mentioned, or list key features to seek in the mass I just described. Or, it may suggest an evidence-based recommendation for follow up of a small lung nodule I just detected.[212,213] Structured reporting facilitates this real-time decision support for the radiologist, a novel technology that will revolutionize how radiologists work in the years to come.

Reuse of Report Information

Let's face it, once a radiology report has been read by the referring clinician (assuming it was read at all), it is rarely used again. A text report is not useful for subsequent research. In contrast, structured reports are "database-able." Once report information is available in electronic form, report data can be used to examine and improve clinical processes, measure compliance with accreditation and certification requirements, profit from federal performance incentives, and enhance participation in imaging research.

For example, I am eager to know how often I recommend chest CT relative to my peers for an equivocal finding on a chest radiograph study. I also want to know how often the chest CT studies I recommend reveal clinically significant abnormalities. These measures track my performance, similar to call-back rate and yield for mammographers. Performance feedback based on structured reporting makes all radiologists better by identifying radiologists who should be emulated and radiologists who need additional training.

Effect on Productivity

Productivity is the elephant in the room. If structured reporting could be obtained at no cost, but nevertheless slowed radiologists down, it would still face serious adoption challenges. Radiologists interpret between 30 and 300 studies per day, depending on case mix. A technology that adds 30 seconds of interpretation time per case adds between 15 minutes and 2½ hours to a radiologist's day. Or, considered another way, lower productivity reduces a radiologist's earning potential by $12,500–$125,000. That's real money, and explains much of the resistance to adopting these systems.

Early PACS faced resistance for the same reasons: clunky technology that slowed radiologists down and required expensive equipment and high-cost personnel. Early PACS mimicked how we interpreted images, often by using eight monitors, four over four, each displaying 15 cross-sectional images in a three by five grid, just as they had been printed on film. We soon realized that only two display monitors were needed and that cross-sectional images could be displayed in cine mode, accelerating interpretation times and improving accuracy. New reporting technologies may soon get over this technologic hump with equivalent innovations.

Structured Reporting: What Your Practice Can Do Today

If you are persuaded that some form of structured reporting should be adopted in your practice, what can you and your practice do *today*? As we wait for new reporting options to emerge, we must use current systems and standards to make our reports more consistent and useful, with minimal impact on radiologist efficiency. Below are some of the low hanging fruit.

Adopt Standard Report Headings

It's surprising how radiologists become attached to relatively insignificant aspects of their reports. Some radiologists prefer *Impression*, others prefer *Summary*, and a small minority believes in *Conclusion*. Advocates for each group can feel quite strongly. Likewise, some radiologists believe the Summary section should come first, whereas others feel it should appear at the end.

Because the stakes involved are quite low, agreeing on standard names and ordering can be a good early exercise to test the waters of standardized reporting in your practice. If you and your colleagues can agree on standard report headings, you certainly will make it easier for human report readers, including other radiologists, who are frequent consumers of radiology reports. If your practice partners cannot reach consensus, remember that computers understand synonyms and can easily reorder sections that have standard names. It's surprising how this single small step can open the flood gates of change.

Tip: For the naming of sections, call on a higher authority to generate a consensus. Consider starting with the RSNA Structured Reporting Committee and its consensus master template.[109] (See Chapter 6.)

Standardize Templates to Ensure Regulatory Compliance

Certain elements of the report are the subject of legislation or are important for certification, which can be a strong driver of adoption. The first standardized reporting tools introduced into my practice were practice-wide templates that assisted us in complying with these mandates. For example, our billing compliance office required attending radiologists to attach an attestation statement to reports dictated by trainees. A standard template makes this task less burdensome.

Agree:

> ATTENDING RADIOLOGIST AGREEMENT:
> I have personally reviewed the images and agree
> with the preliminary report without modification.

The Joint Commission requires that radiology practices approve a list of critical results, document communication of each critical result, and monitor compliance with the documentation policy. The first step toward an optimal critical results policy is to standardize how those results are reported, so notification information can easily be extracted automatically. In my previous practice, departmental policy required the use of the following template for all result communications.

Notification:

> RESULT NOTIFICATION: [These observations] were
> communicated to and acknowledged by [provider
> name] at [time] on [date]. [ ]

Because this template had a consistent format, it was paired with a business intelligence tool to create a compliance dashboard like the one shown in Figure 50.

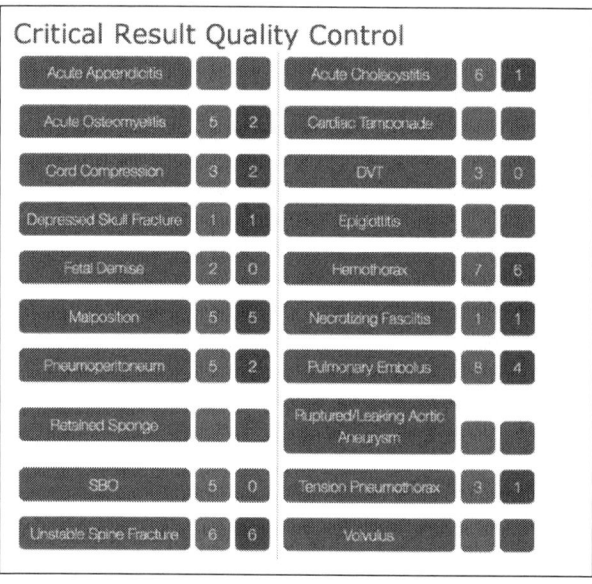

Figure 50. A dashboard created to show the status of critical test results that have not yet been communicated to the clinician. (Reproduced with permission from Montage Healthcare.)

Track Discrepancies between Trainees and Faculty

As an academic practice, my former colleagues and I used a coordinated set of templates to identify the trainee reports that were changed by the attending radiologist the next morning.

Major Change:

```
**ATTENDING RADIOLOGIST CHANGE:
ATTENTION: There are significant changes to the
preliminary report, as follows: [ ]
```

Minor Change:

```
*ATTENDING RADIOLOGIST CHANGE:
I have personally reviewed the images and agree
with the preliminary report, with the following
modifications or additions: [  ]
```

Addition:

```
***ATTENDING RADIOLOGIST ADDITION:
I have personally reviewed the images and agree
with the preliminary report, with the following
additions: [ ]
```

Great Call:

```
***ATTENDING RADIOLOGIST AGREEMENT: I agree with
the preliminary report without modification.
```

Notice the strategic use of asterisks and unique headers, which enabled simple text processing algorithms to identify and track discrepancies between resident and attending interpretations.[214,215] and to notify radiologists automatically via email when a discrepancy statement was missing.

Adopt Common Templates for Divisions and Sections

Can radiologists in your practice agree on what constitutes the best order of findings for ICU chest radiograph reports? Can you agree on a standard order for organs in an abdominal CT report? If so, you could begin creating common templates using current technology. Ideally, a standard order should be developed in consultation with referring clinicians, then given by default to all new members of the practice, including trainees.

Those who embark on a program to standardize reports quickly realize that the main challenges are not technologic, but sociologic.[216] Any form of writing, including radiology reporting, is inherently personal. Patterns of prose develop over many years, often decades. Old habits are difficult to break. And even radiologists who trained together and have practiced in the same environment for years develop different turns of phrase that are as comfortable as an old pair of blue jeans: faded and frayed, but also friendly and familiar. Even the best radiologists find it challenging to adopt reporting patterns that are unfamiliar. And referring clinicians may offer yet another opinion on the optimal fit of a particular report element. But if you can agree on standard templates, the resulting reports will please your customers.

Tip: An easy first step toward structured reporting would be to agree on standard templates for radiology reports across your practice. You will need to allow for differences among studies (diagnostic vs therapeutic, simple vs complex).

Create Selection Lists with Trigger Words

Many current speech recognition systems, including the one I use every day, allow the user to define a template field containing a list of phrases. Each phrase can be selected by a mouse click or by dictating an assigned keyword. Triggering phrases by dictating keywords can be a highly efficient method of reporting, enhancing the consistency of reporting and facilitating subsequent natural language processing.

For example, Figure 51 shows the options for describing the lungs from my default template for chest radiographs. The options listed can be selected by dictating a keyword or phrase to describe the appearance of the lungs on a chest radiograph.

This template took me about half an hour to create, but it has saved me thousands of hours since then. Most observations on a chest radiograph fall into one of these categories. If there is pneumonia, or some other less common observation, I simply dictate my own narrative instead of choosing one of these options. If your reporting system allows pick lists with trigger phrases, it's worth the up-front investment to design a comprehensive list. Your radiology colleagues soon will be asking for a copy.

Keyword(s)	Report Sentence
Clear	The lungs are clear.
Congestion	Mild pulmonary vascular congestion is present. There is no evidence of associated pulmonary edema.
Mild	Mild diffuse interstitial pulmonary edema is present, likely cardiogenic.
Moderate	Moderate alveolar pulmonary edema is present, likely cardiogenic.
Marked	Marked diffuse pulmonary edema and consolidation are present.
Atelectasis	Subsegmental atelectasis is present at both bases.
Left atelectasis	Subsegmental atelectasis is present at the left base.
Right atelectasis	Subsegmental atelectasis is present at the right base.
Effusion	Bibasilar opacities represent small bilateral pleural effusions with overlying atelectasis.
Left effusion	An opacity at the left base represents a small pleural effusion with overlying atelectasis.
Right effusion	An opacity at the right base represents a small pleural effusion with overlying atelectasis.
Everything	Small bilateral pleural effusions are present with overlying atelectasis. Mild cardiogenic interstitial edema also is present.
Low volume	The inspiratory volumes are small, which probably explains increased interstitial opacity and atelectasis at the bases.

Figure 51. Sentences describing lung findings that can be inserted in a report by selecting keywords in my default chest radiograph template.

Use Global Assessments

I recently came across the passage below that describes an adrenal mass in an abdominal imaging report.

```
The mass is probably arising from the right ad-
renal gland, secondary to old trauma. A primary adrenal
cortical carcinoma would be an alternative considera-
tion, although the calcification is usually finer and
more diffuse than this appears. The mass is not clearly
separate from the right kidney, making it difficult to
exclude an exophytic renal mass, but this is less
likely.
```

145

Following this detailed description and erudite differential diagnosis of the lesion, the radiologist makes a recommendation for follow-up.

> `Correlative imaging with MRI may be helpful.`

I suspect this radiologist was hoping to leave the decision about further imaging to someone else. But who is best equipped to make that decision? Is it the primary care physician who ordered the study, who almost never encounters images of adrenal masses? Is it the urologist to whom the patient will probably be referred, who might encounter adrenal lesions more frequently, but who likely has little knowledge of how the subtle imaging features shape the differential diagnosis? Or should the radiologist, who is trained to relate imaging findings to pathologic diagnoses, take responsibility for recommending the next best step in the work-up of this lesion?

Last year, the radiologists from my former practice at the University of Pennsylvania came to the conclusion that the radiologist must assume this role. Radiologists interpreting cross-sectional images began including a global assessment code in each report to represent explicitly the risk of malignancy in solid organs. Any mass in the liver, pancreas, kidneys, or adrenal glands was coded according to the system shown in Figure 52. (See reference [62] for more details.)

> `0: Indeterminate. If indicated within the patient's clinical context, follow up [MODALITY] is advised.`
>
> `1: Benign. No mass.`
>
> `2: Benign. No further evaluation needed.`
>
> `3: Indeterminate. Future imaging follow-up may be needed. If indicated within the patient's clinical context, follow-up [MODALITY] is advised within [TIME PERIOD]`
>
> `4: Suspicious. May represent malignancy.`
>
> `5: Highly suspicious. Clear imaging evidence of malignancy.`
>
> `6: Malignant. Known cancer.`
>
> `7: Benign. Completely treated cancer.`
>
> `99: Cannot be classified. Technically inadequate for evaluation of masses.`

Figure 52. Global assessments used in each abdominal cross-sectional imaging report at the University of Pennsylvania.[62]

For over a year, these codes have been assigned to tens of thousands of reports. Early anecdotal evidence suggests that referring clinicians are delighted to have clear recommendations for each mass. An automated "tickler file" is created to track the patients who require further follow-up, which comforts the risk management office. The data will soon be analyzed to provide feedback to radiologists on the rate at which they assign each code and the chance of malignancy when they assign a code. The data also represent a treasure trove for researchers, who can measure the relationship between imaging features and the chance of cancer, as has been done for breast imaging.[217,218]

As time passes, innovative radiology reporting tools like this one will look more and more like those used for breast image reporting.[176] In the next chapter, we will consider how these tools will affect radiologist efficiency and effectiveness.

Chapter 9:
Standard Terminology for the Radiology Report

When I took the first survey of my undertaking, I found our speech copious without order, and energetick without rules: wherever I turned my view, there was perplexity to be disentangled, and confusion to be regulated.
—Samuel Johnson, in the preface to the first widely used dictionary of the English language

(Note: Portions of this chapter were adapted from references[175–179].)

Lessons from Aviation

Every year, millions of tourists visit the Canary Islands, a small volcanic archipelago off the southern coast of Morocco. On a fateful Sunday in 1977, 380 of those visitors, along with 16 crew members, were aboard Pan Am flight 1736, a 747 jumbo jet that originated in Los Angeles, stopped at JFK airport in New York, and was headed for Gran Canaria Airport.

A second group of 249 passengers and crew were aboard a KLM airlines jet headed from Amsterdam to the same island airport. The plane was captained by an experienced and respected pilot, whose face was featured in the airline's advertising around the world.

At 1:15 PM on that day, a separatist group, opposed to the "colonial occupation" of the Canary Islands by the collapsing government of Generalissimo Francisco Franco, placed a bomb in the airport flower shop that exploded and injured one person. As a result, the airport closed. Inbound planes were diverted to a tiny nearby airport on the northern tip of the neighboring island of Tenerife, blocking its taxiways with planes.

When the Gran Canaria Airport opened a few hours later, the aircraft clogging the Tenerife Airport prepared to make the brief hop to their destination. Because the Tenerife taxiways were full, the KLM plane was instructed by the control tower to "back taxi" down the runway and make a U-turn and wait for takeoff clearance. The Pan Am plane was instructed to follow behind and turn off the runway short of the end. As the two jumbo jets followed each other backward down the runway, a dense fog descended. After the KLM jet completed its U-turn, the planes were face-to-face, half a mile apart.

When the control tower provided flight instructions for "after takeoff," the KLM captain believed he had been cleared. The KLM plane then used a nonstandard and unclear phrase, "at takeoff," to confirm:

KLM #4805: Ah roger, sir, [...]. We are now at take-off.

At that point, the brakes of the KLM plane were released, and engine acceleration became audible on the cockpit voice recorder. Although the plane was rolling for takeoff, the tower believed the KLM aircraft was still waiting for clearance. The tower used a nonstandard confirmation, "OK," and asked the plane to wait for takeoff clearance:

TENERIFE TOWER: OK.... Stand by for take-off, I will call you.

The Pan Am plane, hearing the ambiguous statement from the KLM plane, gave a reminder that it was still on the runway:

PAN AM #1736: And we're still taxiing down the runway, the clipper one seven three six.

Unfortunately, the transmissions from the tower and the Pan Am jet occurred at the same time, resulting in interference in the KLM cockpit that garbled both messages.

The tower then replied by asking the Pan Am plane to confirm when it was clear of the runway.

TENERIFE TOWER: Ah, papa alpha 1736, report the runway clear.
PAN AM #1736: OK, will report when we're clear.

This communication was heard clearly by the flight engineer in the KLM cockpit as it hurtled down the runway, but his concern was dismissed by the captain.

KLM #4805 Flight Engineer: Is he not clear then?
KLM #4805 Captain: Oh yes.

Ten seconds later, desperately trying to avoid the Pan Am plane, the KLM pilots attempt to coax the plane airborne. But its landing gear and engines collided with the body of the Pan Am jet, resulting in 583 deaths, still the deadliest aviation accident ever.

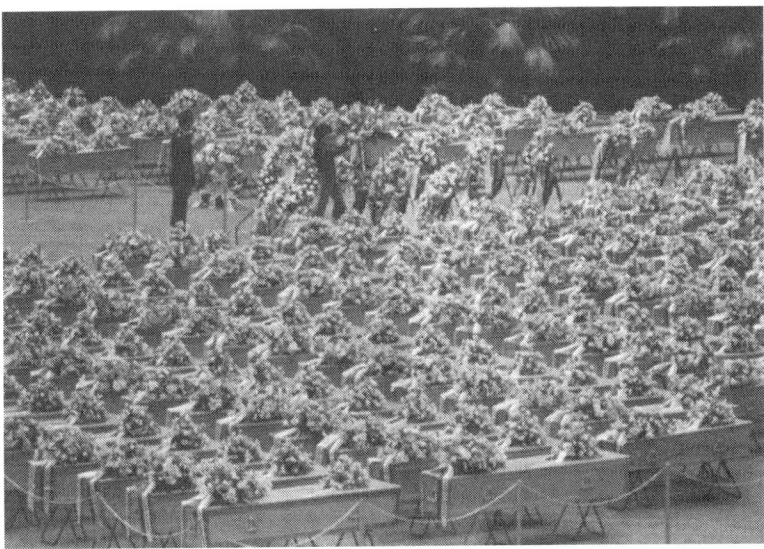

Figure 53. The memorial service for the victims of the Tenerife Airport disaster. (Photo from Nationaal Achief.)

The response of the aviation community to this disaster was swift and sustained. The accident investigation was one of the first to consider the contribution of "human factors" to aircraft accidents.

The specific terminology issues raised by this incident were addressed directly. Today, air traffic controllers no longer use the word "takeoff" in communications to cockpits unless they are giving clearance for takeoff. Instead, aircraft moving into position for takeoff are now instructed to "line up and wait." Any instructions given prior to takeoff use the word "departure" rather than takeoff, to avoid any misunderstanding. And, an emphasis was placed on explicit acknowledgment of communications, rather than simply stating "OK" or "Roger."

In recognition of the team dynamics at play in the cockpit, a program of "Crew Resource Management" was instituted to place more emphasis on team decision making. As a result of these responses, and many other interventions, the rate of fatal airline accidents has decreased dramatically since the early 1980s (see Figure 54).

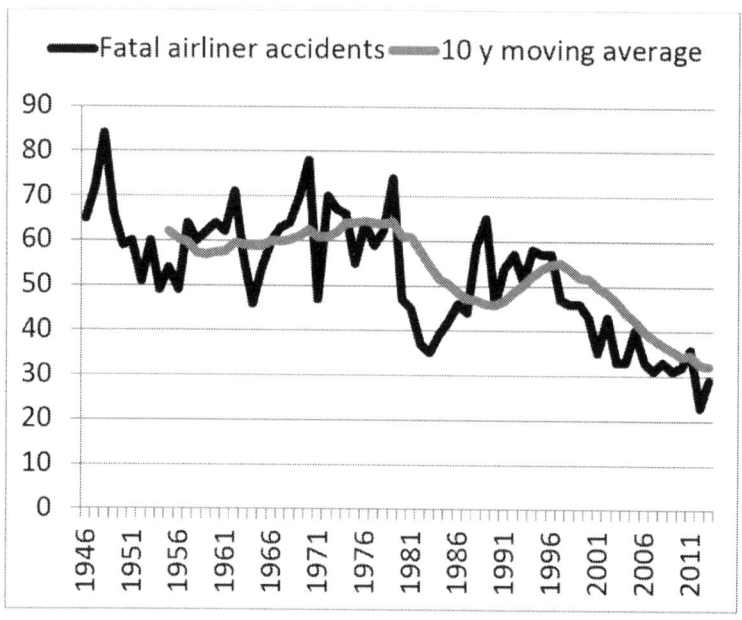

Figure 54. A plot of fatal airliner accidents. The black line shows the number of accidents each year. The gray line shows the 10-year moving average. Accidents began decreasing dramatically after responses to the Tenerife accident were instituted. (Data courtesy of the Aviation Safety Network.[219])

The Tenerife disaster is a story of well-trained professionals doing their best in a life and death situation, with dramatic consequences caused by a constellation of errors, including the use of nonstandard terminology. The parallels to clinical communication are clear, although the consequences of health care failures are sometimes less obvious. Unfortunately, poor communication in radiology probably harms more people every year than the number who died at Tenerife.

BI-RADS: The Advent of Standard Terminology

Decades ago, mammography reports suffered from many communication weaknesses—what the American Medical Association (AMA) called "unintelligible descriptions and ambiguous recommendations."[220] Breast imagers have since put their communication issues behind them, just like the aviation industry. The development and implementation of the ACR's Breast Imaging Reporting and Data System (BI-RADS®) can serve as a template for other areas of radiology, for which the AMA's critiques still ring true today.

By now, BI-RADS is almost universally known—radiologists have used it routinely for over 2 decades to express the information in breast images as actionable conclusions for referring providers. The leaders who developed BI-RADS saw the radiology report as a weak link in the process of caring for women with breast disease. They began by defining the overall structure of a breast imaging report, which until then had contained only prose narrative with inconsistent word choices. Next, they established a set of clearly defined terms for breast imaging observations, including recommended descriptors based on objective evidence of discriminatory power. To further clarify the descriptors, an atlas was soon developed to help radiologists recognize when a given descriptor was present. Then BI-RADS "final assessment categories" were devised to represent a small set of actionable conclusions, oriented toward decision making. These categories are now attached to all breast imaging reports and have become one of the most important and widely known elements of BI-RADS. As with other medical terminology, the BI-RADS terms have been refined and improved over time based on evidence from the published literature. As a result, BI-RADS has become a de facto standard terminology, not only for clinical breast imaging, but also for the research that advances the care of breast disease.

BI-RADS Benchmarking

In conjunction with the breast lexicon and atlas, the BI-RADS committee established a framework for data collection and auditing, which now includes the National Mammography Database (NMD). The NMD aggregates data from multiple breast imaging practices to develop benchmarks for quality. By tracking BI-RADS categories and relating them to patient outcomes, a radiology practice now can inform its radiologists when their practice patterns differ significantly from those of local colleagues or national norms. Thus, the BI-RADS initiative, together with the NMD and other ACR programs, can be viewed as part of a comprehensive approach to improve breast imaging and breast image reporting, rather than merely as a lexicon, an atlas, or a reporting system.

Assessing BI-RADS

BI-RADS has produced many concrete benefits to radiologists, referring clinicians, and patients: It provides clear definitions of breast imaging terms and a visual atlas of salient imaging features that correlate with breast disease. It serves as an important template for the consistent teaching of breast image interpretation, which now can readily convert novice radiologists into expert breast imagers.[221] And it has yielded benchmarks for many essential process and outcome variables, such as call-back rates for screening examinations and cancer rates for each BI-RADS category.[222,223]

While the story of BI-RADS yields many encouraging lessons, it also reveals the pitfalls and unintended consequences of structured reporting. Although BI-RADS focuses on the communication of information from radiologists to their referring colleagues, most radiologists today receive inadequate clinical information about the studies they are asked to interpret.[127] Radiologists cannot produce clinically relevant reports without an accurate and detailed clinical context in which to render an interpretation.[124] As we address radiology communication issues, improvements must be made in both directions on this two-way street.

The BI-RADS experience also sheds light on what many view as an unfortunate accompaniment to this impressive initiative: federal legislation. The Mammography Quality Standards Act (MQSA) required radiologists to attach BI-RADS codes to each report before technologic systems were available to automate that process, creating inefficiencies and adding costs. Modern structured reporting systems now readily create databases to track data on radiologist performance and satisfy MQSA requirements. But requirements of the MQSA still impose significant costs on breast imaging practices, which must purchase structured reporting systems and hire the staff to maintain and use them.

In the coming months and years, radiologists face an unprecedented opportunity to promote the full potential of imaging by including clear and actionable clinical information in all radiology reports. Pay-for-performance initiatives and patient-centered care processes are already prompting us to reexamine our communication methods, which often fail to convey the insights gained from the images we produce every day. The MQSA experience also suggests that problems with communication should be addressed well before they become a key focus of policy makers and legislators. As we consider the challenges of radiology reporting, BI-RADS represents a tested and successful approach that could be applied across all radiology subspecialties to standardize, measure, and improve the process of radiology communication.

Although BI-RADS is the best known and most widely used standard reporting language, several dictionaries and glossaries have been produced by other subspecialty groups to improve the quality of reports for other disorders, including lower limb venous disease,[224] brain arteriovenous malformations,[225] lumbar disk pathology,[226] and chest disease.[98] The ACR itself has recently followed the successful BI-RADS blueprint to foster the development of reporting terminology in other areas of radiology, including LI-RADS for liver lesions,[141] HI-RADS for traumatic brain injury,[143] Lung-RADS™ for lung cancer screening,[227] and PI-RADS to improve early diagnosis and treatment of prostate cancer.[142]

RadLex: Clinical Terminology for Radiology

As the language in the radiology report becomes more consistent, an acute need arises for sources of standard terminology. In the later stages of installing the eDictation reporting system described in Chapter 8,[193] we discovered we had just such a problem. The system was designed to provide choices for the radiologist based on a hierarchical terminology. For a knee MR imaging report, the system needed a list of the anatomic structures a radiologist might describe and a list of the observations that might be made about each structure. BI-RADS terms were available for the breast but what about other areas of radiology? (The other -RADS terminologies pertain only to certain narrow anatomic areas, and in any case were not yet available at the time.)

We found that the most complete and widely used medical terminologies developed outside radiology, such as SNOMED-CT,[228] could not adequately represent much of the information in a radiology report.[194] Likewise the ACR Index, which was a widely used system to organize film-based radiology teaching files by anatomy and pathology, had significant limitations in the electronic world.[229]

To satisfy eDictation's insatiable need for terminology, I became a nonstop terminology developer. But the process was unsustainable for a single individual. This difficult experience convinced me of the need to create a nonproprietary consensus standard terminology to represent the content of radiology reports. I was fortunate to find others who held the same view on the Radiology Informatics Committee of the RSNA. We proposed that the

RSNA establish the RadLex® terminology to serve as a single unified source of terms to represent information in radiology reports.[230]

RadLex was designed to help radiologists standardize key elements of their reports, link report information to the EMR, and retrieve data from teaching files and research repositories. Unlike earlier terminology systems for imaging, RadLex is designed for use in software applications.

In spring 2003, 12 radiologists convened to consider the first draft of thoracic anatomy terms. Following this successful pilot, the RadLex terminology development effort began in earnest in 2005. In the first year, six lexicon development committees each met twice to review and approve anatomic terms and pathologic terms. Two years later, six additional committees were recruited, each focusing on a specific imaging modality. The modality committees met to review, discuss, and approve terms that describe attributes of the devices, imaging exams, and procedure steps performed in radiology departments.

The structure of RadLex approximates the model for describing imaging observations we discussed in Chapter 2. For example, Figure 55 below shows the RadLex term corresponding to key elements of an observation in a radiology report.

Report Element	RadLex® Clinical Term Categories
Observation	Imaging observation, pathophysiologic finding
Anatomic location	Anatomic entity
Modifiers	RadLex® descriptor
Uncertainty	Certainty descriptor

Figure 55. RadLex clinical terms, available at http://radlex.org, are organized according to an information model similar to the model for radiology observations discussed in Chapter 2.

In the end, over 150 expert radiologists, physicists, and other domain experts participated in the creation of RadLex. Approximately 12,000 terms were released publicly in conjunction with the annual meeting of the RSNA in 2007. The lexicon now contains tens of thousands of terms and is freely available from the RSNA.[230] As a result, today we have a relatively complete lexicon to represent the content of radiology reports.

The RadLex Playbook

The RadLex committees next turned their attention to cataloguing all the studies that can be performed in a radiology department, affectionately called the RadLex *Playbook*,[231] a list of all the "plays" we can "call" in a radiology department. (Betsy Humphries of the National Library of Medicine first suggested this sports metaphor.) The RSNA assigns attributes to each exam code to signify modality, body region, anatomic focus, administration of intravenous contrast material, and many other characteristics of the study.

The first and best customer of the Playbook initiative was ACR's Dose Index Registry (DIR), which aimed to track and benchmark radiation exposure by CT exam type across the country.[232] The leaders of the ACR registry effort had a problem: How can radiology practices be measured against one another when their names for the same CT study were completely different? Out of necessity, the first version of the Playbook became a cooperative effort between the ACR and RSNA to standardize CT study descriptions.

When the ACR registry received a new CT study description, the ACR worked with RSNA to assign values for each attribute of the study. ACR and others soon had submitted hundreds of CT descriptions. RSNA developers automatically checked the attributes of each new term to determine if they matched an existing Playbook code or if a new code needed to be created. A simple algorithm gave a name to each new Playbook code. A few codes from the resulting set are shown in Figure 56.

RPID	Letter Code	Short Description	Long Description
RPID2	CTABCA	CT Abd Angio w/wo	CT Abdomen Angio w and wo IV Contrast
RPID3	CTABU	CT Abd wo	CT Abdomen wo IV Contrast
RPID4	CTABC	CT Abd w/wo	CT Abdomen w and wo IV Contrast
RPID5	CTABE	CT Abd w	CT Abdomen w IV Contrast
RPID6	CTCHCA	CT Chest Angio w/wo	CT Chest Angio w and wo IV Contrast
RPID7	CTHDCA	CT Head Angio w/wo	CT Head Angio w and wo IV Contrast

Figure 56. A sample of the RadLex® Playbook version 1. The short and long descriptions were generated automatically from the attributes of the codes.

These Playbook codes worked well for the ACR DIR, because all submitted studies with the same modality, body region, and mode of intravenous contrast agent administration mapped to the same Playbook code, even if the descriptions from disparate radiology practices were different.

Unfortunately, this "crowd-sourced" version of the Playbook could not meet the needs of most other practices. Attributes assigned to submitted descriptions were inconsistent. For example, some coders assumed that an unspecified mode of administering intravenous contrast material meant none was given, whereas others assumed it represented a generic code that allowed the radiologist to decide. As a result, the Playbook became bloated with a panoply of exam codes that many practices did not want to adopt.

At the University of Pennsylvania, we encountered this problem first hand when we planned to use the Playbook as a tool to unify exam codes across multiple facilities. The bloated term database prevented us from using the first version. Instead, we used a consistent methodology to assign attributes to the codes at each of our facilities based on discussions with our local experts. We knew that when we submitted each facility's codes to the RSNA, the assigned RSNA Playbook code would match whenever our assigned attributes matched. Thus we used Playbook codes to cross-match disparate but semantically identical codes across all our facilities to create a single usable set.

The automatically generated names in the original Playbook posed an additional problem. Many found its electronically generated names difficult to parse, particularly for more complex exams. Consider "MG BREAST GUIDE ADD AR SM BD RG CYST LT ASP." It doesn't roll off the tongue. As part of the University of Pennsylvania harmonization process, we used a consistent methodology to assign more intuitive descriptions to each code manually. We also created short strings of letters for each code that many organizations use in their systems. Figure 57 shows how this process unified six disparate codes into a single unified code.

This unified code set is now available for download on the RadLex Playbook web site (http://playbook.radlex.org) as the "Core Playbook." RSNA is currently working to include these codes in a nationally sanctioned terminology for laboratory orders and results, called Laboratory Observations, Identifiers, Names, and Codes (LOINC),[233] and to harmonize the information models for the two terminologies. The result will be a national standard for radiology orders and results.

Org	Exam Code	Description in RIS
A	HEXC	ct head combined
B	HCTC	CT HEAD/BRAIN W/WO CONT
C	ct003	70470-CT Head Unenhan & enhanced
D	CTHD2	CT Head with and without contrast (70470)
E	CTHD2	CT Head with and without contrast (70470)
F	ct203	70470-CT HEAD, W/WO CONTRAST-TUTTLEMAN

Performing Orgs	Exam Code	Description in RIS
A, B, C, D, E, F	CTHDC	CT Head w & wo IV contrast

Figure 57. The conversion of multiple comparable radiology exam codes to a single RadLex Playbook code. In this example, codes with the same meaning from six different facilities are converted to a single unified code.

The Benefits of RadLex

RadLex (and terminology work in general) is like plumbing. Very few users of plumbing know or care how the pipes work; they simply want the toilet to flush when they push the handle. The early developers of RadLex laid the water mains and feeder pipes, built drainage systems, and established standard fittings to supply radiology with its vocabulary. But most radiologists have limited interest in the details of pipe laying and trench digging.

Now that RadLex is widely adopted, it quietly permeates many aspects of radiology practice. Listed below are some of the many benefits of RadLex clinical terms and the RadLex Playbook.

Structured reporting templates. —The RSNA report templates described in Chapter 8 use RadLex codes to link radiologist's observations to the EMR, the images themselves, and a wide variety of reporting and decision support tools.

Imaging order entry decision support. — ACR appropriateness criteria can be triggered automatically because imaging studies are described by standard terms.

Consistent image display protocols. — Because imaging studies have consistent names, launching a study from the work list results in consistent image display.

Default template selection. — Speech recognition systems can identify the modality and body region from a Playbook code, enabling them to display the correct default template automatically.

Decision support for the radiologist. — Decision support tools can recommend vital information automatically for the radiologist,[234] triggered by standard terms in the radiology report. For example, these tools can assist radiologists in following evidence-based guidelines, can alert radiologists to possible diagnoses, and can retrieve relevant information from PubMed, the Internet, or proprietary decision support databases.

Creation of image libraries. — Standard terms in the radiology report can be used to retrieve the imaging study from a teaching file or other image library.

Data retrieval and data mining. — RadLex makes report search more accurate. RadLex synonyms enable a search for "renal stone" to retrieve reports mentioning "kidney stone" or "urolithiasis." And search for "lung" and "cancer" can retrieve reports describing "adenocarcinoma in the right upper lobe."

Registry reporting and benchmarking. — A key purpose of registries is to benchmark across practices. Practices submitting registry data with Playbook codes attached are ensured of receiving apples-to-apples comparisons.

Specifying imaging protocols. — When a radiologist or technologist receives an order for an imaging study, a plan for the appropriate sequence of procedure steps, commonly called an *imaging protocol*, is needed. RadLex Playbook codes facilitate automation of the protocol selection process.

Intelligent prefetching. — Many PACS implementations store older images in less accessible storage, requiring prefetch of prior studies relevant to a scheduled patient's upcoming exam. Playbook codes enable accurate determination of relevance through direct comparison of Playbook attributes, such as modality and body region.

As the RadLex clinical terms and the Playbook become more widely adopted, more of these benefits will become apparent in daily practice. Samuel Johnson, one of the earliest lexicographers of the English language, defined a lexicographer as "a humble drudge." As an increasing number of our information systems have "RadLex inside," we can thank the many humble drudges who made it possible.

Chapter 10:
How to Think about Imaging Information

True genius resides in the capacity for evaluation of uncertain, hazardous, and conflicting information.
—*Sir Winston Churchill*

(Note: Portions of this chapter were adapted from reference [235].)

As we interpret clinical images, we form an interconnected network of ideas in our head—about the relative location of findings, about the progression of a pathophysiologic process, and about how imaging features suggest the presence or absence of disease. This network of thought, which underpins the radiology report, stands in stark contrast to the inherently linear form of the report: a string of words with a beginning, a middle, and an end.

In this chapter, we examine the fundamental underpinnings of clinical decision making—an indispensable foundation for thinking about imaging information and creating a convincing narrative report. For the radiology report to be optimally understood, the reasoning process that led to its conclusions must be especially clear.

To animate this material, which is inherently mathematical, we will become acquainted with several gentlemen whose work over the past few centuries provides a model for thinking and decision making. Insight into their underlying motivations helps to illustrate how their theories apply to the practice of radiology reporting. And their stories of discovery mirror the reasoning processes that imaging professionals go through every day.

Logic and the Radiology Report

Professor George Boole and Logical Inference

I speak here [of] mathematics in its larger, and I believe, truer sense, as universal reasoning expressed in symbolical forms, and conducted by laws, which have their ultimate abode in the human mind.
—George Boole

George Boole grew up in the early 1800s as the son of a struggling shoemaker in a small industrial area near Sheffield, England.[236–238] Although shy throughout his life, George excelled in elementary school and supplemented his education by helping his father build cameras, kaleidoscopes, microscopes, sundials, and telescopes. His formal schooling ended there, but he became a locally renowned child prodigy for his self-taught classical language and calculus skills, which led to a junior teaching position at the age of 16, a gold medal from the Royal Society for an early mathematical treatise, and ultimately, at the age of 34, the first professorship in mathematics at Queens College in Cork, Ireland.

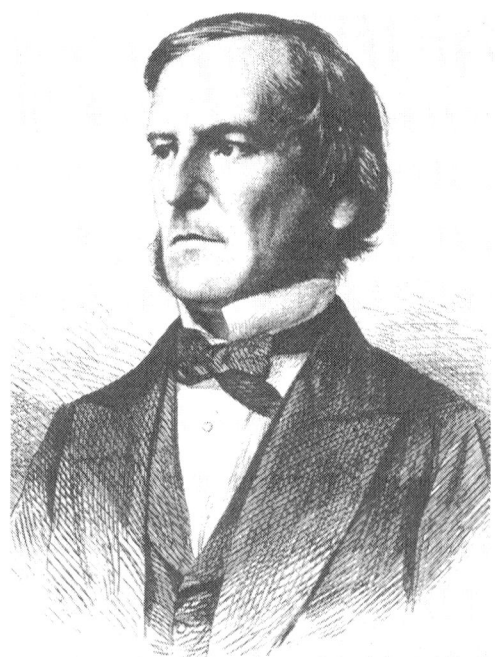

Figure 58. George Boole, the father of modern logical analysis.

Just 2 years later, Professor Boole had become Dean of Faculty and posed the following question at his annual address:

...whether there exist, with reference to our mental faculties, such general laws as are necessary to constitute a science.[239]

Thus began his attempt to identify "those universal laws of thought which are the basis of all reasoning." (Clearly, he was an ambitious man.) His subsequent treatise on the topic, "An Investigation of the Laws of Thought, on Which Are Founded the Mathematical Theories of Logic and Probabilities,"[240] was published in 1854, when he was 38 years old.[236] This mathematical analysis of logical inference established Boole as the father of modern logical analysis and, ultimately, one of the pioneers of computer science.

Boolean Logic

Boolean logic deals with *propositions*—essentially simple statements of fact. For example, "a mass is present in the left lower lobe" is such a statement. Or, to borrow a famous proposition from Aristotle, "all men are mortal."

Boole's system of logic rested on a fundamental assumption: Each statement must be either absolutely true or completely false. The beauty of Boole's system is that all manner of wonderful conclusions can be drawn from a set of propositions according to simple *logical operators*. For example, the operators, OR, AND, and NOT, can combine propositions to infer new facts.

Figure 59 below shows the commonly used Boolean operators, which take on the meaning you would expect from common use.

A	B	NOT A	NOT B	A AND B	A OR B	A NOR B	IF A THEN B
T	T	F	F	T	T	F	T
T	F	F	T	F	T	F	F
F	T	T	F	F	T	F	T
F	F	T	T	F	F	T	T

Figure 59. A summary of Boolean algebra. For example, the first row in the chart shows that if A is true and B is true, then the proposition A AND B must also be true. A OR B is true if either A or B is true. NOT A is true only if A is false, and so on.

Despite Boole's early death at the age of 49 from "an attack of fever, ending in suffusion on the lungs" (or as we might say today, "a pneumonia with parapneumonic effusion"), Boole's insights had a profound and lasting impact on subsequent mathematical thought and, ultimately, on many aspects of life, including the computer and the radiology report.

For example, when scientists built the first computers in the late 1930s, they recognized that Boole's true/false logic readily applied to the on/off nature of a binary circuit. Today, computer chips are fabricated from millions of miniscule electronic logical components, called "gates," arranged according to Boole's tenets. Some of the earliest computer programs that displayed "artificial intelligence" were inference engines that created logical proofs using Boolean principles, systematically drawing new conclusions from an initial set of facts using these fixed rules of logic.[241]

Boolean Logic Applied to the Radiology Report

The beauty of logical inference is its simplicity and believability, making it ideal for intuitive rhetoric and persuasion in human speech. When scientists first began to describe the way humans think, whether about medical evidence or about the mortality of man, they began with Boolean logic.

A common form of logical inference, first popularized by Aristotle, is called the syllogism. With apologies to Aristotle:

All men are mortal.

This patient is a man.

This patient is mortal.

How might we apply Boolean logic to the information in a radiology report? For example, a radiologist may believe that when two imaging observations, A and B, are present, disease C is also present. This is simply a form of the Aristotelean syllogism:

All patients with observation A and observation B have disease C.

This patient has observation A and observation B.

Therefore, this patient has disease C.

But wait a minute! To apply logical inference to patient care, each piece of medical evidence and each clinical conclusion must be either 100% true or 100% false. No uncertainty. No hedging. In the real world, and especially in radiology, uncertainty abounds. Those attempting to apply Boolean logic to medical inference quickly discover that imaging observations seldom definitively confirm or exclude a diagnosis on their own. And radiologists often disagree, not only on the final diagnosis, but also on whether particular imaging features are present.[136,137]

A syllogism that more closely mirrors radiology inference would stump both Boole and Aristotle, and might look more like this:

All men may be mortal.

He is probably a man.

Is he mortal?

Unfortunately, when uncertainty is present, Boole's rules of logic no longer assist us.

Probability and the Radiology Report

Reverend Bayes and Updating Uncertain Belief

The shortcomings of logical inference were first contemplated in the 1700s, ultimately leading to new insights relevant not only to the radiology report, but also to a vital recreation of the time, gambling. For example, if a jar contains five black marbles and 95 white marbles, the chance of drawing a black marble is 5%; if we draw a card from a deck, the chance it will be an ace is 4/52, because four of the 52 cards are aces. These gambling questions put probability to practical use. Any gambler whose probabilistic thinking was not well calibrated soon became a pauper.

In medicine, the best parallel to the deck of cards is the published literature. Journal articles often supply data about the frequency of important events, such as the survival rate for patients with cancer or the rate at which an imaging observation is present in patients with a particular disease. For example, if 72 of 191 patients with invasive ductal carcinoma have a spiculated mass on breast MR images, the probability that a spiculated mass will be observed in a patient with breast cancer is 72 /191, or 38%.[218]

And yet, at the time of diagnostic imaging, we often do not know whether the patient has breast cancer; we only know whether a spiculated mass is present. We may start with an opinion, or pretest belief, about the likelihood of breast cancer based on the evidence thus far. The radiologist must determine how that pretest belief should change based on the presence of a spiculated mass.

The answer to the radiologist's conundrum requires a more sophisticated and practical form of reasoning than simple Boolean logic. The Reverend Thomas Bayes proposed just such an inference method.[242,243] Bayes' work provided clear mathematical rules for probabilistic inference, directly analogous to the forms of logical reasoning described by Boole but applicable to *uncertain* propositions.

Little is known about Bayes' life, but as a young man, he enrolled at the University of Edinburgh to study logic and theology. He soon became a Presbyterian minister, which allowed him plenty of time for his avocation: thinking and writing about mathematics.

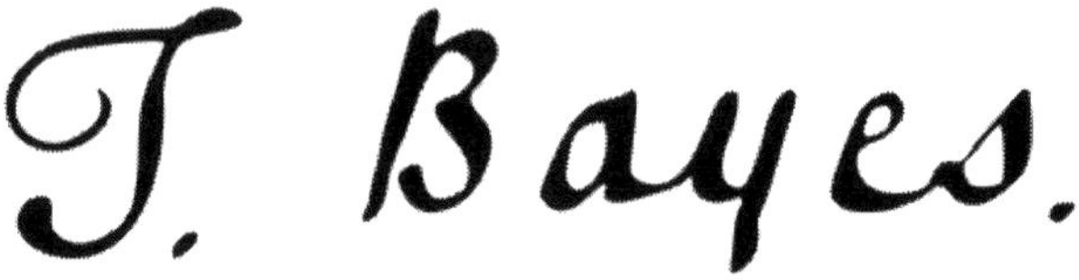

Figure 60. The signature of the Reverend Thomas Bayes, who first expressed a key mathematical rule for probabilistic reasoning. There are no known portraits of Bayes, so his appearance is uncertain. (Perhaps that is fitting….)

Although Bayes' key findings on probability were never published during his lifetime, the colleague who facilitated their posthumous publication was motivated by his desire to confirm "the existence of Deity".[242,244] He asked: Given that certain events occur in the world, what is the likelihood that a Deity has caused those events? This line of inquiry elucidated the crux of all forms of diagnostic testing—what was then called the "inverse probability" and what we now call Bayes' theorem or Bayes' rule.

Marquis de Laplace Makes Probabilistic Reasoning Practical

Bayes' work remained in obscurity until Pierre Simon de Laplace, a brilliant French contemporary of Bayes, recognized its applicability to a wide variety of practical problems. Laplace was born into a well-to-do family of farmers and cider traders just across the English Channel from Bayes, near the north coast of Normandy, France.[245] An impressive student, at age 16 he was sent by his father to study theology at a nearby university. Instead, he fell in love with mathematics and 3 years later left for Paris to study with a preeminent mathematician, Jean d'Alembert.

d'Alembert asked Laplace to address the burning question of the day: Newton's theory of gravitation had moved the sun to the center of the solar system, but the heliocentric theory did not precisely match the astronomic observations of the time. Many thought the solar system was unstable and that Jupiter would soon crash into the sun.

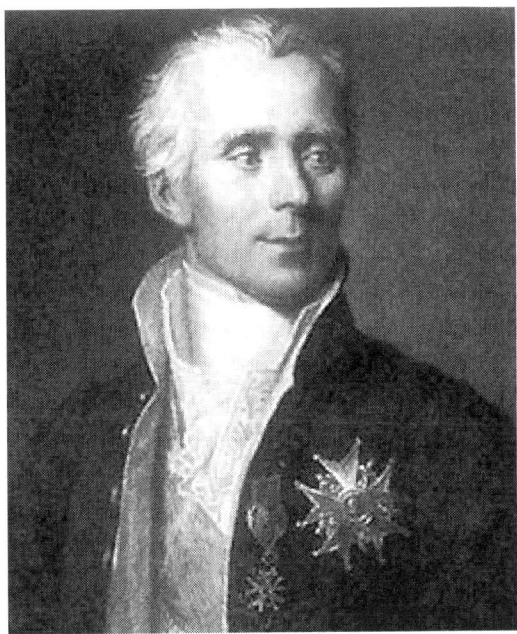

Figure 61. Pierre Simon de Laplace, who first conceived modern methods of probabilistic reasoning.

After trying several approaches to explain the astronomical observations, Laplace had a key insight: The imprecision of the observations themselves was the problem, not Newton's theory. Thus began Laplace's interest in uncertainty and his search for quantitative methods to understand the true nature of things, based on a set of observations.

Laplace reached young adulthood just as Thomas Bayes' work was first published in an obscure English-language journal. (You might say it had a low impact factor.) Laplace probably never read Bayes' original essay, but he clearly had read many of the same treatises that Bayes studied. Ten years after the publication of Bayes' essay, Laplace's "Memoire on the Probability of the Causes of Events"[246] elucidated the key mathematical underpinnings of Thomas Bayes' work and showed how it could be put to practical use.[247,248] One of the seven principles enumerated at the beginning of LaPlace's essay was:

When two events depend on each other, the probability of the compound event is the product of the first event and the probability that, this event having occurred, the second event will occur.

Or, restated as a clinical example: The probability of having both breast cancer and a positive breast MR imaging study is equal to the probability of a positive breast MR imaging study multiplied by the chance of breast cancer when the breast MR imaging study is positive. The following simple equation mirrors Laplace's principle: P(A and B) = P(B) x P(A given B).

Another of Laplace's principles was:

If we calculate a priori the probability of the occurred event and the probability of an event composed of that one and a second one that is expected, the second probability divided by the first will be the probability of the event expected, drawn from the observed event.[246]

Illustrated clinically: The probability of having both breast cancer and a positive breast MR imaging study is equal to the probability of breast cancer multiplied by the chance of a positive breast MR imaging study when cancer is present. Here is a mathematical expression of that statement: P(A and B) = P(A) x P(B given A).

Perform a little algebra (Hint: set the two equations equal to one another using P(A and B)), and we derive what today we call Bayes' rule (Figure 62).

$$p(A \text{ given } B) = \frac{p(B \text{ given } A) \times p(A)}{p(B)}$$

Figure 62. Bayes' theorem of probabilistic inference. We often refer to P(A) as the prior probability, P(A given B) as the posterior probability, and P(B given A)/P(B) as the "evidential support" B provides for A.

This equation is at the core of all diagnostic decision making. It revolutionized how we draw conclusions based on uncertain evidence. Using this key insight, Laplace went on to elaborate the application of Bayes' theorem to numerous real-world questions, including the movements of Jupiter and Saturn, the veracity of witnesses, the gender mix of French children, judicial decisions, voting, and myriad games of chance.

Whether they know it or not, radiologists apply the same inference methods: The published literature tells us how often patients with breast cancer exhibit a given observation on MR imaging studies. Bayes' theorem tells us how to calculate the reverse quantity, which has more clinical utility: the probability of cancer in a woman whose MR imaging study exhibits that observation.

Subjective Probability: It's All in Your Head

Initially, Laplace analyzed events whose frequency could be counted and measured. But he also recognized the limitations of this approach, because the probability of many important events is difficult to measure. His landmark essay concluded with this lament:

> *The irregular events of nature are not exactly comparable to the drawing of the numbers of a lottery. Thus, chance has no reality in itself. It is nothing but a term for expressing our ignorance of the way in which the various aspects of a phenomenon are interconnected and related to the rest of nature.*[246]

Laplace was acknowledging the limits to what is now called a "frequentist" view of probability.[249] For example, to determine the chance that a flight will leave on time, a frequentist would look at the airline's web site to determine exactly how often its planes had departed on time in the past. But veteran air travelers know there are more nuanced questions: What is the likelihood of on-time departure when the forecast calls for thunderstorms? Or when the plane is flown by a particular pilot? Perhaps we also should consider the specific aircraft and its maintenance record. As with clinical medicine, we rarely have statistics for the exact combination of conditions that are actually present.

Typically, we ask expert prognosticators to adjust the known frequentist statistics (e.g., overall percentage of on-time departures) based on expert judgment. To set the appropriate odds, judgment must take into account all of the relevant data. The strength of this "subjectivist" view is its reliance on the wisdom of an expert decision maker who has weighed all the evidence, including empiric frequentist statistics such as the on-time percentage.

The essence of subjective Bayesian decision making is the notion that probabilities are simply a means to measure our belief in uncertain propositions. For radiologists and other clinical diagnosticians, the question is: Given the imaging observations and other clinical data, what is the chance that the patient has the disease? Diagnosticians recognize that a probability estimate is a belief that should be informed by the best current observations, whether from large data sets, expert opinion, or other life experiences. Therein lies what distinguishes great radiologists: their ability to layer evidence from the published literature over their vast experience to form a differential diagnosis. The foundational work of our statistical forefathers turns out to have immense practical utility for radiologists today. Boole, Laplace, and Bayes would be gratified.

Reasoning under Uncertainty and Diagnostic Imaging

Bayesian principles can help answer another key question radiologists face every day: What is the most appropriate imaging test for a particular patient? Consider the following clinical scenario: A referring physician asks you about the results of a diagnostic mammogram you interpreted yesterday. In the upper outer quadrant of the left breast, you identified a cluster of suspicious microcalcifications—not the kind that suggest definite cancer, but those that indicate the need for a more definitive diagnosis. The referring physician relays the patient's desire to consider a breast MR imaging study. How would you decide whether that study is right for that patient? If the MR imaging results were negative (or positive), how would you use them to help make the decision whether or not to perform a biopsy?

The answers to these questions are derived from Bayesian reasoning, as well as evidence from the radiology literature, and calculated measures of diagnostic accuracy, such as sensitivity, specificity, predictive values, and receiver-operating characteristic (ROC) curves. These measures can seem abstract, but to apply evidence from the clinical literature, radiologists need to know: Which descriptors of a test are the best intrinsic measures of performance? Which are the most clinically important? What are the weaknesses of sensitivity and specificity? What do ROC curves represent? Why are predictive values clinically relevant, and what are the pitfalls associated with their use? A basic understanding of these concepts, which we will now review, is vital to the appropriate utilization and reporting of diagnostic imaging studies.

Pearson's Two-by-Two Table: A Simple Tool

Whether phenomena are qualitative or quantitative, a classification leads to a contingency table, and from such a table we can measure the degree of dependence between any two phenomena.
—Karl Pearson

Karl Pearson is one of the fathers of what today we call "statistics." An English mathematician, Pearson founded the world's first statistics department at University College London in 1911. Like many great scientists, he carefully studied the works of his scientific forebears, including Laplace.[250]

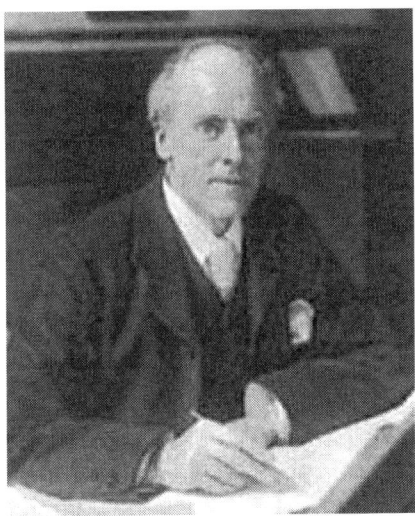

Figure 63. Karl Pearson, an English mathematician who is widely viewed as the father of modern statistics.

Pearson's contributions to statistics include early work on correlation, *p*-values, the Chi-squared test, and many other enduring concepts.[251] Pearson's profound influence on the science of radiology arose from his description of an intuitive method to analyze diagnostic tests: the two-by-two table, which Pearson called a "contingency table."[252] This deceptively simple device can be jotted on the back of an envelope but nevertheless is versatile and powerful in understanding test accuracy.

Figure 64 illustrates the prototypical form of Pearson's two-by-two table, applied to a diagnostic imaging test. Across the top, we see two columns: One contains all cases (patients) in which the disease is truly present (D+), and the other contains cases in which the disease is truly absent (D−). Along the left side of the table, we see the two possible test results: positive (disease presence, T+) and negative (disease absence, T−).

	D+	D−	Totals
T+	TP	FP	TP+FP
T−	FN	TN	FN+TN
Totals:	TP+FN	FP+TN	N

Figure 64. A two-by-two "contingency" table describing diagnostic test performance.

The table illustrates the relationship between the test result and the presence of disease and defines four different table "cells." In the first row, we see that a positive test result can be either a true positive (TP) or a false positive (FP), depending on whether the disease is present or absent.

The second row shows that a negative test result can be either a false negative (FN) or a true negative (TN), again based on whether the disease is present or absent. (Note: Sometimes false positives are called "alpha" or "type I" errors and false negatives are called "beta" or "type II" errors. I find it difficult enough to remember TP, TN, FP, and FN, much less to keep track of Greek letters and numbered types, so I avoid those latter notations altogether.)

The beauty of the two-by-two table is what it reveals about the performance of the test: The first column of the table displays how the test performs on patients who have the disease in question. The second column specifies how the test performs on patients who do not have the disease (or who are "normal" with respect to the disease in question). At the bottom of each column, the total number of patients who actually do and do not have the disease is listed.

A total of the first row, at the far right, shows the total number of patients who had positive test results; the second row total indicates the number of patients who had negative test results. An overall total at the bottom right indicates the total number of patients who participated in this study of test performance (N).

We must acknowledge that Pearson's two-by-two tables require certain simplifying assumptions when applied to diagnostic imaging. The first assumption is that the test in question must be compared with a reference standard that specifies the truth about the presence or absence of the disease (D+ or D− in Figure 64). In the past, this standard commonly was called a "gold standard," a term that is falling out of favor, perhaps because many reference standards are imperfect. For example, even clinical diagnoses supplemented by the best histopathologic techniques are fallible.[253]

A second major assumption of the two-by-two table is that the test result must be considered either positive or negative (T+ or T− in the table above). This is perhaps the least appealing assumption, since many tests have continuous values, such as the degree of stenosis in a vessel or the attenuation of a liver lesion. (We will reexamine this assumption when we discuss ROC curves.[254–256])

Our final simplifying assumption is to assess test performance with respect to the presence or absence of a single disease and not several diseases.

The Two-by-Two Table Applied to a Radiology Test

Figure 65 contains data from an actual experiment to evaluate the accuracy of breast MR imaging in patients with clinically or mammographically suspicious lesions. All patients had suspicious lesions and were about to undergo tissue sampling, just like the patient we described above. Before biopsy, each woman underwent contrast-enhanced MR imaging of the breast. The histopathologic examination of the specimen obtained from a subsequent excisional biopsy was used as the reference standard for disease. (Note: I recognize there are many more diagnostic and therapeutic options available after a positive mammogram today, but we will simplify this example by considering only an open biopsy. A more detailed description of the experimental methodology and a reporting of the final data can be found in reference [257].)

	Malignant	Benign	Totals
MRI+	71	28	99
MRI-	3	80	83
Totals:	74	108	182

Figure 65. A two-by-two contingency table showing actual patient data from an experiment to study breast MR imaging.

A grand total of 182 women were enrolled in the study at the time the table was constructed. Of those, 74 had cancer, and 108 did not. There were a total of 99 positive test results, 71 true positives and 28 false positives. The 83 negative test results were composed of three false negatives and 80 true negatives.

Tip: The two-by-two table is a simple tool that summarizes how a diagnostic test performs.

Sensitivity and Specificity

Important probabilistic measures of test performance can be computed from the two-by-two table. *Sensitivity* and *specificity* are the most popular methods for describing the accuracy of a diagnostic test and are widely used throughout the clinical literature.

Sensitivity: Probability of Disease Detection

Sensitivity measures how well a diagnostic test performs on *patients who actually have the disease* in question. We compute sensitivity by using the numbers in the first column of the two-by-two table in Figure 65. *Sensitivity* represents how often the test will find the disease when it is present, or TP / (TP + FN).

Of the 74 women who actually had cancer, 71 had a positive MR imaging study. Thus, the sensitivity of breast MR imaging in the sample of women undergoing breast biopsy is 71/74. Stated another way, 96% of women with cancer were identified by MR imaging.

Tip: Sensitivity measures how a diagnostic test performs in a population of patients who have the disease.

Specificity: Correct Identification of "Normal" Patients

Specificity concerns the ability of a test to give an appropriately negative result in *patients who do not have the disease*. *Specificity* is defined as how often a normal patient will have a normal test result, or TN / (FP + TN).

Specificity is calculated by using the numbers in the second column of the two-by-two table (see Figure 65). Of the 108 women who had benign lesions, 80 had negative MR imaging studies. Thus, the specificity of breast MR imaging in the sample of women undergoing breast biopsy is 80/108, or 74% of women without breast cancer will be identified as such by MR imaging.

Tip: Specificity measures how a diagnostic test performs in a population of patients who don't have the disease (i.e., "normal" patients).

Which Is More Important: Sensitivity or Specificity?

How can sensitivity and specificity be used to determine whether a test is useful in a specific clinical situation? Sensitivity and specificity are important measures, but which is more important? The woman with the suspicious breast mass can help us clarify these questions. How we would feel if we were to miss a cancer due to a false-negative study? Because we would regret this outcome, there is an appropriate emphasis on developing and enhancing the sensitivity of breast MR imaging to avoid missing cancers that may progress after a false-negative study.

We also would feel uncomfortable about sending a patient for an excisional biopsy of a benign lesion, but perhaps less so, since this result would occur even if MR imaging had never been performed. Thus, the main beneficial role of breast MR imaging in this setting is to allow some women without cancer to avoid an excisional biopsy. We therefore can conclude that sensitivity is more important than specificity in this clinical setting. For a quantitative discussion of how these principles operate, see reference [258].

Tip: A sensitive test is more valuable in situations where false negatives are more undesirable than false positives. A specific test is more valuable in situations where false positives are more undesirable than false negatives.

Limitations of Sensitivity and Specificity

Sensitivity and specificity are important descriptors of a diagnostic test because they do not vary greatly among patient populations. (See reference [259] for some exceptions to this rule.) But the woman with a suspicious lesion on her mammogram wants to know whether breast MR imaging can help her. Now that we have computed sensitivity and specificity from a two-by-two table, we can tell her the following: "If you have cancer, the chance that the MR imaging study will detect it is 96%. If you don't have cancer, the chance that the MR imaging study will be normal is 74%." These statements are often difficult for patients and health care providers to incorporate into their clinical reasoning because the statements are focused on the test, not on the patient. The patient and the referring clinician are left to figure out how they apply. Thus, a key weakness of sensitivity and specificity is that they are not immediately relevant to clinical decision making. So measured sensitivity and specificity convey little that helps us assess a test's optimal clinical role.[260]

An additional weakness of sensitivity and specificity is that the two quantities cannot always be used to rank the accuracy of two tests (or two radiologists). This weakness is particularly evident when one test has a higher sensitivity but a lower specificity than another.

The reason test-comparison difficulties arise with sensitivity and specificity is that the two quantities are inherently related: You cannot evaluate one without the other. As sensitivity increases, specificity tends to decrease and vice versa. We see this principle every day when we see two colleagues who interpret the same images differently. Consider how two radiologists decide whether congestive heart failure is present on a chest radiograph. One reader may use strict criteria for congestive heart failure, calling fewer positives, thereby lowering sensitivity and raising specificity. The other reader may employ more lax criteria, calling more radiographs positive for congestive heart failure, thereby increasing sensitivity but lowering specificity. In this situation, it is impossible to determine whether one radiologist is better than the other from comparisons of sensitivity and specificity alone.

Tip: Sensitivity and specificity of a diagnostic test are related to one another and have limited utility for specific clinical decisions.

ROC Curves: Comparing Diagnostic Tests

The United States first faced the limitations of sensitivity and specificity during World War II. The exigencies of the war led to an intense interest in radar detection of enemy aircraft—a task quite similar to detecting disease on medical images. Military personnel watched a screen called a radar receiver, looking at blips and attempting to classify them as enemy, friend, or false signal. Military commanders noticed that the accuracy of radar-receiver operators varied widely.

In 1944, General Eisenhower sent a team of engineers to the European theater of operations to check the radar equipment that would be used during the D-Day landing. The team found nothing wrong with the radar equipment but noticed an interesting pattern among the human operators. When the true-positive results were plotted against the false-positive results, the radar-receiver operators tended to fall along a consistent curve. The curves captured the strict or lax detection behavior of each reader (favoring false positives or false negatives) and came to be known as "receiver operating characteristic" curves or ROC curves. The name stuck; the rest, as they say, is history.

The team Eisenhower sent to Europe included Lee Lusted, the son of a Methodist minister from Mason City, Iowa.[261] After his trip, Lusted attended medical school at Harvard, completed a radiology residency at the University of California, San Francisco, and became a radiologist. Recognizing the similarities between the decisions made by radar-receiver operators and radiologists, he became one of the pioneers in the use of ROC curves in radiology and medicine. (Before he died in 1994, I had the honor of meeting Dr. Lusted, a brilliant, wonderful, and gentle man who took special interest in junior scientists.)

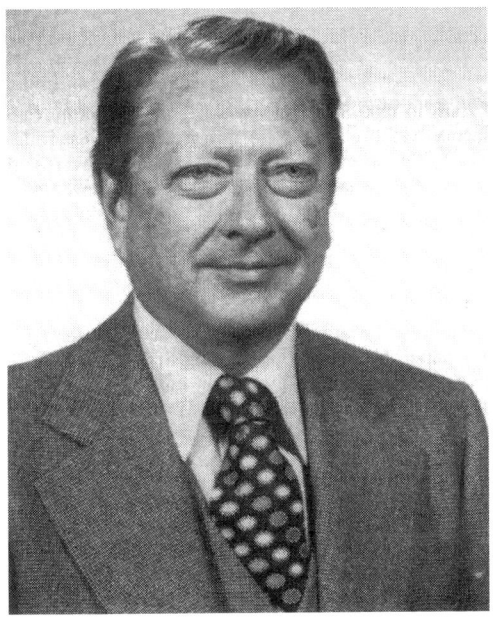

Figure 66. Lee Lusted, a radiologist who first applied ROC
curves to medical diagnostic tests.

Dr. Lusted recognized that ROC curves held the answer to a few key questions in radiology: When one test is more sensitive, but another is more specific, how should we decide which test provides better diagnostic information?[262] Or are they really quite similar, except that one test uses stricter criteria for a positive result?

Lusted's ROC curves answer these questions. By relaxing the assumption that a test must have only two values, positive and negative, he imagined the readers of these two imaging tests specifying their results on a rating scale.

Figure 67 shows a six-point rating for the identification of breast cancer on images. This scale asks the reader to specify one of the six categories: definitely cancer, likely cancer, possibly cancer, possibly benign, likely benign, and definitely benign.

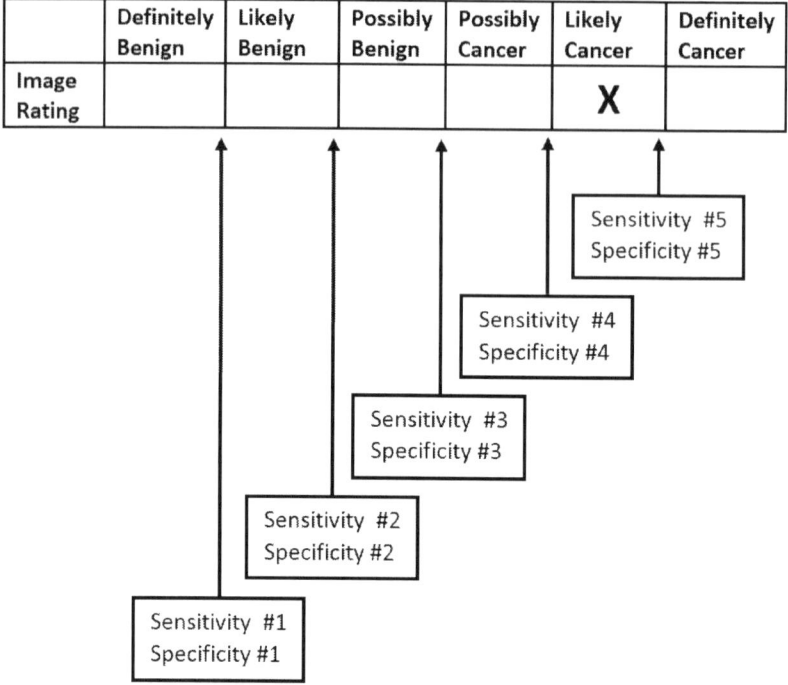

	Definitely Benign	Likely Benign	Possibly Benign	Possibly Cancer	Likely Cancer	Definitely Cancer
Image Rating					X	

Figure 67. A six-point scale for rating the presence or absence of breast cancer. Placing a cutoff between rating categories creates two-by-two tables from which sensitivity and specificity can be calculated.

The ratings then are tabulated using the two-by-six table shown in Figure 68. The rating scale, and the table it produces, provide multiple opportunities to measure sensitivity and specificity. Assuming the test is "positive" only when "definitely cancer" is selected, and negative otherwise, produces a single two-by-two table. By assuming that the top two ratings, "likely cancer" and "definitely cancer," represent positive test results and that the remaining ratings are negative, a new two-by-two table is formed that yields a higher sensitivity and a lower specificity than the first (because less strict imaging criteria were used and more studies were rated as positive). Repeating this process creates five two-by-two tables, the last of which considers only the "definitely benign" ratings as negative; the remaining ratings are considered positive. The two-by-two table shown in Figure 68 shows this last analysis, which yields a high sensitivity and a low specificity.

	Defi-nitely Benign	Likely Benign	Possi-bly Be-nign	Possi-bly Cancer	Likely Cancer	Defi-nitely Cancer	To-tal
Cancer Cases	2	3	5	10	30	50	100
Benign Cases	50	30	10	5	3	2	100
Totals	52	33	15	15	33	52	200

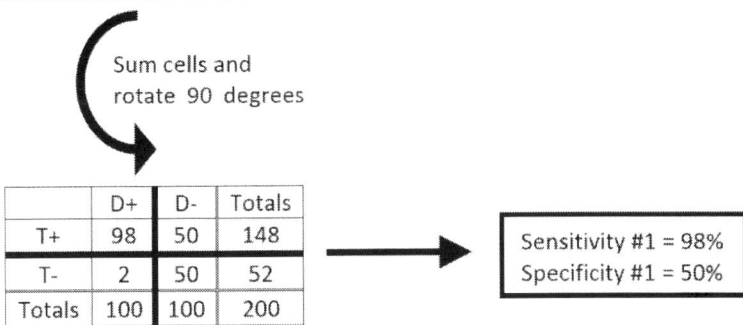

Sum cells and rotate 90 degrees

	D+	D-	Totals
T+	98	50	148
T-	2	50	52
Totals	100	100	200

Sensitivity #1 = 98%
Specificity #1 = 50%

Figure 68. The two-by-six table (top) shows the results of an ROC study of a breast cancer imaging technique. The two-by-two table (bottom) is created by placing a cutoff between the ratings of "Definitely Benign" and "Likely Benign."

Figure 69 shows a plot of all five sensitivity-specificity pairs derived from the two-by-six table in Figure 68. The (0,0) point and the (1,1) point are included to represent the situation in which all images are considered negative or positive, respectively. Some have suggested calling this a *sensitivity versus specificity* curve. Dr. Lusted and the other statisticians who originally created the first curves preferred to model them with an increasing function, so it is conventional to flip the x-axis of a sensitivity versus specificity curve to create an ROC curve (see Figure 70).

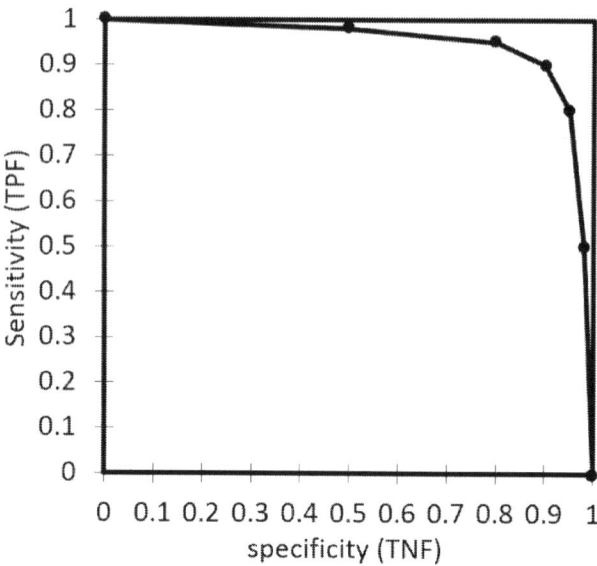

Figure 69. A sensitivity versus specificity curve is a plot of sensitivity versus specificity. (TPF = true-positive fraction, TNF = true-negative fraction.)

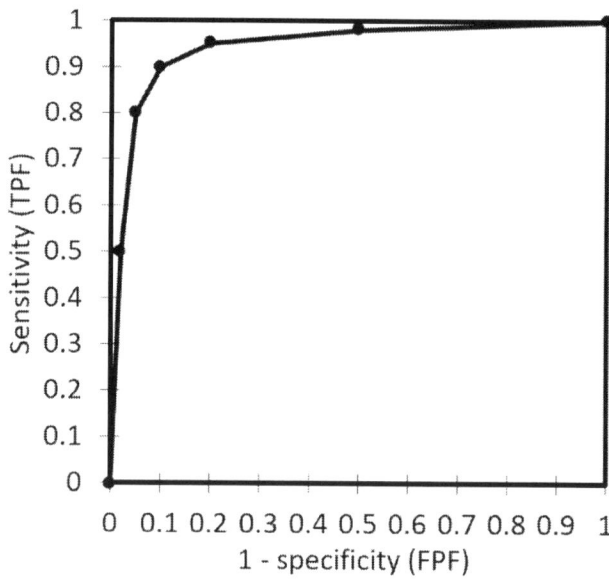

Figure 70. An ROC curve is a plot of sensitivity versus specificity, except that the x-axis has been reversed. (TPF = true-positive fraction, FPF = false-positive fraction.)

ROC curves explicitly represent the inherent relationship between a test's sensitivity and specificity.[263] ROC curves are designed to capture the overall information provided by an imaging test, regardless of how the images are interpreted by a radiologist. Therefore, ROC curves specifically address situations in which tests cannot be compared on the basis of sensitivity and specificity alone. (See reference [255] for a detailed discussion of ROC methodology.)

Tip: ROC curves provide a method to compare diagnostic test accuracy, independent of the diagnostic criteria (strict or lax) that are used.

Clinical Limitations of ROC Curves

How can an ROC curve be used to quantitatively assess the accuracy of a test? The most popular method is to measure the area under the curve, often called A_z, or "A sub z." In general, the larger the area under the ROC curve, the better the diagnostic test. But despite their advantages for research and analysis, ROC curves aren't useful for clinical decision making. The value of A_z has no intrinsic clinical meaning. Should our patient with an abnormal mammogram be satisfied when she learns that the area under the ROC curve for breast MR imaging was 0.83? Unfortunately, there is no A_z value above which (or below which) we can be certain of a diagnostic test's clinical value.

Tip: While ROC area is helpful in comparing two tests, it has limited value to clinical decision makers.

Predictive Values: How Likely Is the Disease?

We have established that sensitivity, specificity, and ROC curves provide an incomplete picture of the clinical utility of an imaging test. But two other quantities have much greater clinical relevance and intuitive appeal: the predictive values.

The two by two table in Figure 65 shows that the probability of cancer in women with suspicious mammograms is 41% (74/182). Thus, simply because she has been referred for excisional biopsy (without knowing the specific mammographic appearance of the lesion), the patient's chance of cancer being present is about 41%. How does the MR imaging result modify the likelihood of cancer to assist clinical decision making? The predictive values answer this question and emphasize an important principle of diagnostic testing: A diagnostic test causes a change in our belief about the likelihood that disease is truly present.

Positive Predictive Value

Positive predictive value (PPV) is defined as the probability of disease in a patient whose test result is abnormal, or TP / (TP + FP). The positive predictive value can be computed by using only the numbers in the first row of the two-by-two table in Figure 65. Ninety-nine patients had positive MR imaging studies. Of those, 71 actually had cancer. Thus, the positive predictive value of breast MR imaging is 71/99, or 72% of the women with a positive MR imaging study have cancer. These quantities are sometimes called post-test probabilities of disease, because the predictive value simply reflects the probability of disease after the test result is known. The positive predictive value tells us that a positive breast MR imaging study raises the probability of disease from 41% to 72%—as we would expect, a positive test result increases the likelihood of disease.

Tip: Positive predictive value indicates the likelihood of disease given a positive test result.

Negative Predictive Value

The negative predictive value (NPV) is the reverse analog of positive predictive value. *Negative predictive value* can be defined as the probability that disease is absent in a patient whose test result is negative, or TN / (FN + TN).

Thus, the negative predictive value can be computed solely from the quantities in the second row of the two-by-two table in Figure 65. Eighty-three patients in our sample had negative MR imaging studies. Of those, 80 actually had benign lesions; there were three false-negative results. Thus, the negative predictive value of breast MR imaging is 80/83, or 96% of women with a negative MR imaging study don't have cancer. (Note: It is simply coincidence that the sensitivity and the negative predictive value are approximately equivalent in this case.) The probability of disease after a negative test result is simply the negative predictive value subtracted from 100%, or 4% in this case. This computation tells us—as we would anticipate—that a negative test result decreases the probability of disease, in this case from 41% to 4%.

Tip: Negative predictive value indicates the likelihood of no disease given a negative test result.

Clinical Utility of Predictive Values

The clinical utility of the predictive values is best illustrated by the first question our patient might ask after she has an MR imaging exam or a biopsy: "Do I have cancer?" In the uncertain world of medicine, we should translate this question as "How likely is it that I have cancer?"

The predictive values, in contrast to sensitivity and specificity, answer these relevant questions and, therefore, are immediately applicable to the clinical decision-making process. When a patient knows that a negative MR imaging study will decrease her chance of having cancer to 4%, several vital questions can be considered by the patient and her doctor: Is a 4% likelihood low enough that biopsy could be deferred during a short period of follow-up? Is it worth trading the potential harm of tumor progression during short-interval follow-up for the potential benefit of not having to undergo excisional biopsy? These tradeoffs are routinely considered by referring physicians, patients, and other clinical decision makers and can be modeled explicitly using techniques we will discuss in Chapter 11. (See reference [264] for a breast imaging example.)

Limitations of Predictive Values

Despite the substantial clinical utility of the predictive values, they are critically dependent on the pre-test probability, or the prevalence of disease in the imaged population. As we learned above, a diagnostic test causes a *change* in belief about the likelihood of disease. As you might expect, the higher the pre-test probability of disease, the higher the post-test probability of disease. So predictive values are directly dependent on the population to which a test is applied.

To illustrate the dependence, consider the following question: Could MR imaging be used as a screening tool to detect cancer in asymptomatic women? This approach has some intuitive appeal, since breast MR imaging is a highly sensitive test and might reveal a greater number of cancers than would be detected at screening mammography.

To examine the implications of this policy, we will simulate what would occur if a group of asymptomatic women were screened with MR imaging. We will represent the incidence of cancer in a screening population with the incidence of cancer for an average-risk 50-year-old woman, which is approximately 0.25%, much lower than in the cohort of women represented in Figure 65. For computational simplicity, we will consider a screening population of 20,050 women, 50 of whom have occult cancer.

Since MR imaging is 96% sensitive, 48 of the 50 women who actually have cancer will have positive MR imaging studies (50 x 96% = 48). The other two women will have false-negative MR imaging studies and will have undetected cancer, just as if they had never undergone screening MR imaging. Based on the 74% specificity for breast MR imaging computed above, 14,800 women will have normal MR imaging studies (20,000 x 74% = 14,800). The remaining

5,200 women will have false-positive studies. A two-by-two table containing these data is shown in Figure 71.

	Malignant	Benign	Totals
MRI+	48	5,200	5,248
MRI-	2	14,800	14,802
Totals:	50	20,000	20,050

Figure 71. Patient data from a hypothetical group of 20,050 asymptomatic women undergoing screening breast MR imaging.

The true disease status for these women will be unknown at the time of testing. Thus, clinical inferences must be drawn from the test results and the predictive values. As we discussed above, the negative predictive value indicates the clinical implications of a negative test. Since there are 14,802 women with negative tests, only two of whom have cancer, the negative predictive value is 0.01% (2/14,802). This represents a decrease from 0.25% and has no real clinical significance (although it has some potential reassurance value).

Figure 72 summarizes our reasoning. There are 5,248 women in our simulation population with positive tests, 48 of whom actually have cancer. This represents a positive predictive value of approximately 1% (48/5,248). Thus, a positive MR imaging study increases the likelihood of cancer from 0.25% to 1%. Unfortunately, this group presents a logistical dilemma. Are we willing to perform 100 biopsies to find one cancer? Probably not. Should these women be followed by a more intensive imaging regimen, such as more frequent follow-up MR imaging studies? Possibly, but the wisdom of such a program is questionable. It would cost tens of millions of dollars and lead to a substantial increase in the number of negative excisional biopsies.

An analysis of this hypothetical screening program shows vast differences in the predictive values of breast MR imaging for a population of women with suspicious mammograms compared with a screening population with a much smaller prevalence of disease. Use of breast MR imaging as a screening test for normal-risk women is highly questionable, whereas the use of MR imaging for women in other populations with higher risk of cancer makes sense. (See reference [265] for another, somewhat dated, clinical example of this phenomenon.)

Despite their limitations, predictive values can be determined mathematically from sensitivity, specificity, and prevalence. Because sensitivity and specificity are often published, a referring clinician can compute the predictive values for a particular population of interest by using the prevalence from that population and the sensitivity and specificity from the literature.

Tip: Positive and negative predictive values are useful for clinical decision making but may vary depending on the population to which a test is applied.

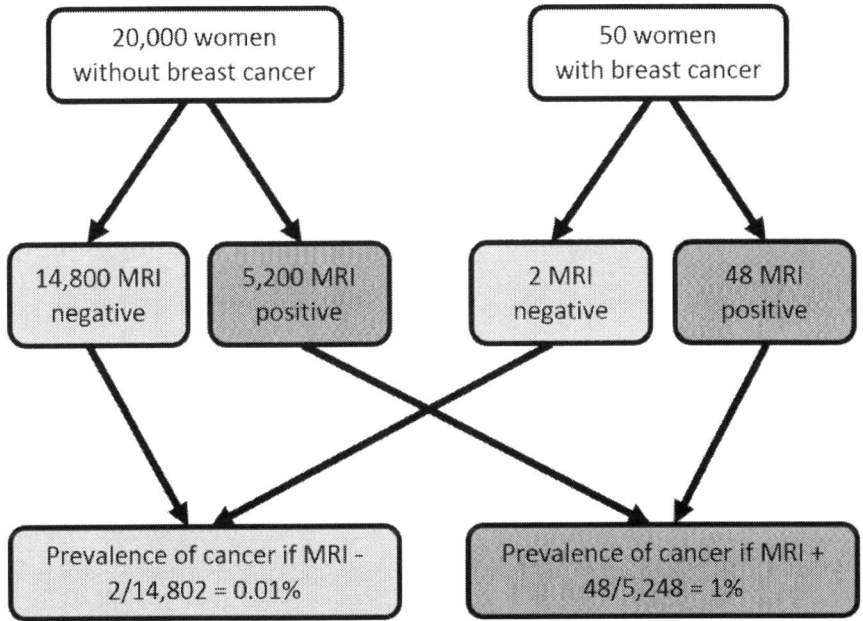

Figure 72. A simulated population of 20,050 women screened with breast MR imaging. The assumed prevalence of cancer in a screening population is 0.25%, approximated here by 50 women with cancer and 20,000 women without cancer.

Likelihood Ratio: Measuring Change in Probability

A somewhat less intuitive concept called the likelihood ratio (LR)[266,267] has many of the advantages of sensitivity, specificity, and predictive values with few of their drawbacks. The likelihood ratio is both unaffected by disease prevalence and can yield clinically useful information. The *likelihood ratio* for a positive test result (LR+) is defined as the likelihood (or probability) that a person with disease would have a positive test, divided by the likelihood that a person with no disease would have a positive test. This quantity is equivalent to sensitivity divided by 1 minus specificity. (Although I promised to limit use of Greek letters, I must inform you that this concept is sometimes referred to by the Greek letter lambda λ.) (Note: There is also a negative likelihood ratio (LR−), which we will not discuss here; it is analogous to LR+.)

LR+ = sensitivity / (1 − specificity).

To illustrate the use of the likelihood ratio, consider the breast MR imaging example: The sensitivity of breast MR imaging is 96% and the specificity is 74%. Therefore, the positive likelihood ratio is 0.96 / (1 − 0.74), or 3.7.

Once the likelihood ratios for a test are known, they become an elegant and simple tool. They can be used to calculate the post-test probability of disease given the pre-test probability of disease. This calculation requires the conversion of probabilities of disease to *odds* of disease. The odds of disease are defined as the probability that disease is present divided by the probability that disease is absent:

Odds(D+) = p(D+) / p(D−).

The odds correspond precisely to how we think about gambling. For example, if there is an 80% chance disease is present, the odds of disease are 80% divided by 20%, or 4:1, which is expressed simply as an odds of 4.0. Likewise, if there is a 20% chance of disease, the odds are 20% divided by 80% or 1:4, expressed as odds of 0.25.

Practical Value of the Likelihood Ratio

The value of converting probabilities to odds and the appeal of the likelihood ratios become clear when calculating the post-test probability of disease. Simply multiply the pre-test odds by the positive likelihood ratio for the test to obtain the post-test odds. For example, the odds of disease given a positive test result is equal to the positive likelihood ratio multiplied by the pre-test odds of disease:

Odds(D+ | T+) = LR+ x Odds(D+).

Finally, to obtain the post-test probability, convert the post-test odds back to the post-test probability, as follows:

P(D+ | T+) = Odds(D+ | T+) / [1 + Odds(D+ | T+)] .

The three formulas above employ the likelihood ratio to calculate the post-test probability of disease from any pre-test probability of disease.

Tip: Likelihood ratios allow quick but nonintuitive calculation of the post-test odds of disease from the pre-test odds.

Limitations of the Likelihood Ratio

The attractive mathematical properties of the likelihood ratio can also cause confusion. For example, likelihood ratios less than 1 indicate a test result decreases the probability of disease; ratios greater than 1 indicate a test result increases disease probability. To many, it is perplexing that a likelihood ratio of 4.0 should increase likelihood to the same degree that a likelihood ratio of 0.25 decreases likelihood. Furthermore, the likelihood ratio only operates on the odds of disease, rather than the more intuitive probability of disease. Some find it counterintuitive that the same likelihood ratio causes different absolute changes in probability, depending on the pre-test probability. And significant expertise is required to apply the likelihood ratio in clinical practice: "The likelihood ratio for breast MR imaging is 3.7; what does that mean for my patient?" Despite these weaknesses, the likelihood ratio remains an elegant tool for analyzing diagnostic tests.

Summary of Tips for Thinking about Imaging Information

1. The two-by-two table is a simple tool that summarizes how a diagnostic test performs.
2. Sensitivity measures how a diagnostic test performs in a population of patients who have the disease.
3. Specificity measures how a diagnostic test performs in a population of patients who don't have the disease (i.e., "normal" patients).
4. A sensitive test is more valuable in situations where false negatives are more undesirable than false positives.
5. A specific test is more valuable in situations where false positives are more undesirable than false negatives.
6. While ROC area is helpful in comparing two tests, it has limited value to clinical decision makers.
7. Positive predictive value indicates the likelihood of disease given a positive test result.
8. Negative predictive value indicates the likelihood of no disease given a negative test result.
9. Positive and negative predictive values are useful for clinical decision making but may vary depending on the population to which a test is applied.
10. Likelihood ratios allow quick but nonintuitive calculation of the post-test odds of disease from the pre-test odds.

Chapter 11:
Decision Making for Diagnostic Imaging

So, when certain maxims are presented for your consideration, you must ask yourself whether you try to behave in accordance with them, or, to put it differently, how you would react if you found yourself violating them.
—Leonard J. Savage

Do radiologists make decisions? You may be surprised to learn that many decision scientists don't think so. These scientists define a decision as an *irrevocable* allocation of resources. For example, a thoracic surgeon must decide whether to perform a pneumonectomy. He can't both perform and not perform a pneumonectomy at the same time; he must choose. Once he performs the pneumonectomy, he can't "take it back". Thus, the surgeon's choice is an irrevocable allocation of time and other resources from the patient, the health care team, and the health insurance company.

Skeptics would say diagnostic radiologists are not decision makers because they just cogitate on the likelihood of disease and assign probabilities. No resources are allocated.

But the process of creating a radiology report, deciding what observations to include, and expressing the likelihood of disease, is at least as difficult as a surgical decision. Assigning a likelihood of cancer to a lung lesion is tantamount to deciding whether an invasive procedure will be performed—certainly irrevocable. Some might say the radiologist's job is even more challenging than the surgeon's, because the radiologist must consider the consequences of all possible decisions that might be based on the conclusions of the radiology report.

Whether a radiologist is a true decision maker or not is relevant only to purists, but it highlights the distinction between assessing likelihood and deciding to act. Regardless of how we answer this abstract question, the principles of decision theory remain essential to the practice of radiology. We will review those principles now.

Blaise Pascal and Decision Making under Uncertainty

There is nothing so conformable to reason as this disavowal of reason.
—Blaise Pascal[268]

Blaise Pascal, a 17th century philosopher and mathematician, drew the connection between likelihood and decision making when considering the following profound proposition: Does God exist?

If I saw no signs of a divinity, I would fix myself in denial. If I saw everywhere the marks of a Creator, I would repose peacefully in faith. But seeing too much to deny Him, and too little to assure me, I am in a pitiful state.[268]

His subsequent analysis of the decision to believe in God, often called "Pascal's Wager," is thought to be one of the first instances of *decision analysis*—a formal quantitative process for determining the optimal decision in uncertain circumstances.

Pascal recognized the essential unknowability of the existence of God. But he also recognized that each individual needed to make a decision that took into account the uncertainty about God's existence—particularly important at a time when it was universally believed that heaven or hell would be part of everyone's real future. Pascal asserted that if God did not exist, the position taken did not matter, but if God did exist, there was "an infinitely happy life to gain" in heaven by believing in the almighty. He decided: "Wager, then, without hesitation that He is."

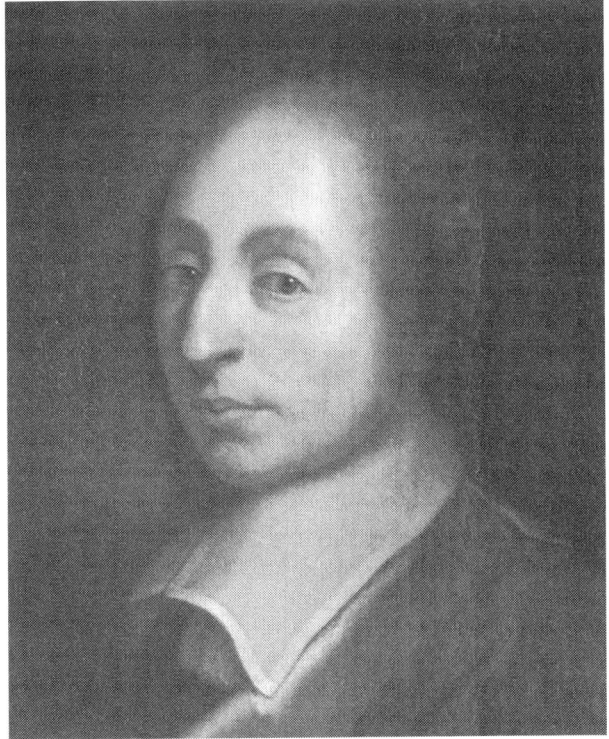

Figure 73. Blaise Pascal, who first described the mathematical relationship between likelihood and values that determines optimal decision making. (Photograph distributed from the Joconde database under a CC BY 3.0 license.)

Pascal's key insight—that multiplying the likelihood of a particular hypothesis by the value we place on its consequences—applies just as well to health care decisions as it does to divinity.

Although we have focused thus far on the role of likelihood in diagnostic imaging, the values we place on the consequences of clinical decisions play an equally important role. Imagine two women with identical risk profiles, and identical MR imaging results, who both end up knowing (based on the predictive value of a negative breast MR imaging study) that they have a lesion in their left breast with a 4% chance of being malignant. Woman #1 cannot bear the thought of living even for a short time with a possibly cancerous lesion in her breast. She decides to schedule a tissue sampling procedure as soon as possible. Woman #2 wants to avoid an uncomfortable and potentially disfiguring procedure and is willing to tolerate temporarily the small risk that a cancer is present. She decides to schedule follow-up imaging in 3 months.

Which woman is correct? In fact, they both are. Two women with the same likelihood of disease can reach two equally correct decisions based on the different values they place on the consequences of their actions.

A New Theory of Decision Making

Laplace and his predecessor Pascal were the first to describe the mathematical relationship between likelihood and values as "the product of the sum hoped for by the probability of obtaining it." This basic principle was later formalized by two brilliant mathematicians, von Neumann and Morgenstern in their 1944 book, *Theory of Games and Economic Behavior*.[269] They showed that if an individual *(a)* had values for various outcomes that could be ranked and *(b)* had beliefs in the likelihood of those outcomes that could be quantified, then the *only* rational course of action was one that maximized the sum of products of the likelihood and value for each outcome. These axioms are intuitive to any gambler. A bet to win $10 if a coin comes up heads is worth about $5 because $10 times 1/2 equals $5.

This new theory of decision making is dependent on a new quantitative notion, called *utilities*. Utilities, which measure the value we place on outcomes, can be intensely personal; there are no right answers. It is no wonder that "shared decision making" has become such a popular notion.[270] Optimal decision making really does require collaboration between the physician, who has the clinical knowledge and experience to estimate the likelihood of various clinical outcomes, and the patient, who is a singular expert on how he or she would feel about those outcomes.

A Clinical Decision Model

To illustrate how the von Neumann-Morgenstern axioms can be used as a clinical decision aid, consider the following scenario (which is admittedly oversimplified). An 80-year-old female patient, who otherwise has a life expectancy of 6 years, has a lung lesion with a 30% chance of being stage I non-small cell lung cancer. She is deciding whether to undergo surgery that has a mortality rate of 10%.

A simple decision tree depicting this decision is shown in Figure 74. The square node indicates a decision between two (or sometimes more) options. Each circular node shows an uncertain event—the outcome of which we can't control and don't know.

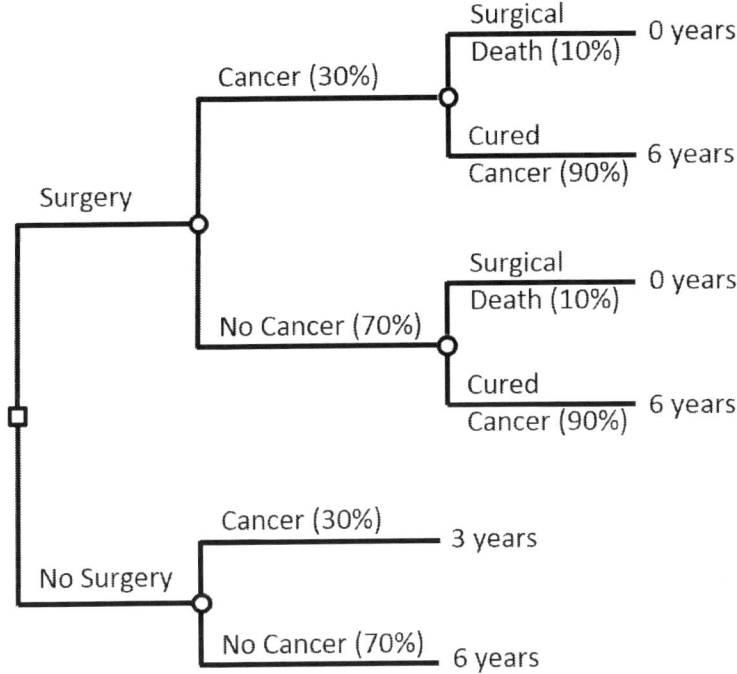

Figure 74. A decision tree depicting the decision whether to undergo surgery for suspected lung cancer. The square node represents a decision. The circular nodes represent uncertainties.

To determine the desirability (often called "expected utility") of each decision option, we apply the same mathematical principles used to value a flipped coin. The expected value of a 90% chance of 6 years of life is 5.4 years (90% times 6). Since we are assuming that surgery always cures the cancer, the expected value is the same whether or not the patient actually has cancer. On the other hand, if no surgery is performed, the patient lives 3 years with cancer and the same 6 years without cancer. The expected utility of this option is calculated by adding 30% times 3 years and 70% times 6 years, for an expected utility of 5.1 years. Therefore, surgery is the preferred option because 5.4 is greater than 5.1.

Such models oversimplify the decision-making process. (The model in Figure 74 is particularly egregious.) But probabilities and utilities are critical for decision making about imaging tests. And these decision aids are an essential foundation of clinical decision making. In fact, an entire science has arisen to construct and refine clinical decision models and manage their underlying assumptions.[271]

Analyzing the Value of Information

Fortunately for radiologists, clinical inference is never conducted with a fixed set of evidence or a fixed set of diagnoses. It is an iterative process, with a cycle of evidence collection, revision of tentative conclusions, and decision making based on currently available evidence. Often, collecting more information is the optimal next step—and that usually means imaging.

Collecting evidence involves a cost, whether it is a dollar cost, such as the cost of a laboratory test or contrast material administration, or the time to interpret the images. Thus, assessing the value of additional information becomes a critical part of clinical reasoning. What is the best next test? Which will be most likely to provide the maximum information? Fortunately, the same rigorous mathematical framework behind decision analysis can also be used to compare the value of information from different diagnostic tests.[272] (We will not review the mathematical framework here.)

Weaknesses of Decision Theory

Decision theory has a strong formal foundation and is empirically useful. Nevertheless, the theory has many critics.[273] Below is a dialog about the limitations of decision theory and the responses that have arisen to address each one.

Weakness: Most people are risk averse and would pay somewhat less than $5 for a coin-flip's chance at $10.

Response: The same is true in clinical decision making—living a shorter time with certainty is often valued more than taking a risk for a longer life. Formal models of risk have arisen to manage risk aversion in finance and can be applied to medical risks as well.

Weakness: Using life expectancy as a utility doesn't consider that a year spent ill with cancer isn't the same as a year spent fully healthy.

Response: To address this shortcoming, many decision models use *quality-adjusted* life years (QALYs), which value years of poor health less than years of good health.

Weakness: Many people value life years differently over time.

Response: Just as the future value of a dollar is worth less than a dollar today, a year at the end of someone's life is not as valuable as a year of life today. Many decision models apply discounts to life years just as banks discount cash flows.

Weakness: Decision models often require data that are not available in the published literature. For example, a mortality rate for stage IV ovarian cancer may be well known, but cancer mortality in a patient with heart disease and multiple myeloma has never been measured.

Response: Bayesians recognize that a probability is simply an expression of belief. When published data are unavailable, models can employ probabilistic estimates from the best experts, who are informed by published evidence.

The critiques are endless. But skeptics of these formal models must also answer the question: What decision-making process should we use instead? Intuition? Experience? The pioneers of decision science, from Pascal and Bayes to von Neumann and Morgenstern, have given us a much more reliable set of tools to inform the clinical decision-making process.

Decision Biases

Whenever there is a simple error that most laymen fall for, there is always a slightly more sophisticated version of the same problem that experts fall for.
—*Amos Tversky* [274]

As a graduate student at Stanford University in the 1980s, I had the good fortune to be in the presence of Amos Tversky on several occasions. Tversky was a humble but brilliant man. His colleagues once joked about the "Tversky intelligence test"—the faster you realized Tversky was smarter than you, the smarter you were.[275] Tversky, in his lifetime collaboration with Daniel Kahnemann, meticulously catalogued the consistent failings of human thought. Over long careers that ultimately led to the Nobel Prize, they showed that humans don't reliably follow the rational decision-making methods we outlined earlier in this chapter.[276]

Natural human modes of behavior, shaped by evolution over millennia, often ignore mathematically optimal decision-making methods. Instead, we tend to rely on intuition that is subject to many human failings. The work of Kahnemann and Tversky has revealed many embarrassing shortcomings of human judgment. They called these decision-making techniques *heuristics*, defined as "judgmental shortcuts that generally get us where we need to go— and quickly—but at the cost of occasionally sending us off course."

While we might hope that lengthy clinical training would make physicians less susceptible to these cognitive biases, much empiric work shows that these biases are equally relevant in medicine and radiology.[277–280] We will now consider a few wild animals in the menagerie of flawed human thoughts that have particular relevance to the practice of radiology.

The Representativeness Heuristic

Representativeness is the degree to which an event is similar to the essential features of a group to which it belongs. In 1973, Kahnemann and Tversky gave the following vignette to experimental participants:

> *Tom W. is of high intelligence, although lacking in true creativity. He has a need for order and clarity, and for neat and tidy systems in which every detail finds its appropriate place. His writing is rather dull and mechanical, occasionally enlivened by somewhat corny puns and by flashes of imagination of the sci-fi type. He has a strong drive for competence. He seems to feel little sympathy for other people and does not enjoy interacting with others. Self-centered, he nonetheless has a deep moral sense.*[281]

Experimental participants were then asked to estimate the likelihood that Tom was a graduate student in one of 10 different fields. Even though participants were given base rates showing that computer science majors were rare, they still ranked Tom as highly likely to be a computer science major because the description was representative of a computer science major. (Note: 40 years later, computer science majors are no longer rare, so this experiment would have a different design today.)

The experiment showed that humans are less likely to incorporate prior probabilities into their judgments than they should. The reaction of physicians to "incidentalomas" follows the same pattern. If the patient has a low prior probability of renal cancer, a small renal mass seen on a lumbar spine MR imaging study is almost certainly a benign cyst. Yet it can be irresistible to pursue a definitive diagnosis with further testing, leading to a cascade of events that can cause serious patient harm.[282] Radiologists and other physicians sometimes try to counteract this tendency by saying "when you hear hoof beats, think of horses, not zebras." We sometimes forget that if the base rate of disease is very low, the chance of disease rises only slightly when an accurate test is positive.

Availability Bias

Availability bias is the incorrect assumption that if examples of an event occur to us easily, the event is more likely. For example, the interest in genetic testing for breast cancer soared after Angelina Jolie announced her decision to undergo prophylactic bilateral mastectomy.[283] As a medical student,

I once visited the student health center for a bump on my knee, thinking I might have an osteosarcoma. Guess what tumors we were studying in class that week... This human failing has a name of its own, "medical students' disease."[284]

For radiologists, a rare disease they saw yesterday can trigger the same erroneous mode of thought—mentioning the zebras before considering the horses.

Anchoring, Framing, and Regret

Anchoring is yet another human failing described by Kahnemann and Tversky. Students were asked to estimate in 5 seconds the product of the numbers between one and eight. Students who were shown the expression 8x7x6x5x4x3x2x1 gave estimates four times higher than those given the ascending sequence 1x2x3x4x5x6x7x8. Their numeric judgments were anchored to the first numbers in the sequence, which affected their estimates accordingly. In analogous fashion, radiologists and other physicians often show illogical resistance to revising their initial diagnostic hypotheses.

Framing of a clinical question can have a powerful effect on subsequent decisions. A lung cancer surgery decision posed in terms of how many patients survived surgery (90%), rather than how many patients died in surgery (10%), was strongly preferred by both physicians and patients.[285]

Regret can cause physicians to inflate the likelihood of events that have an undesirable outcome. So radiologists may overestimate the probability of a diagnosis that they might regret missing.[279] This heuristic may lead to unnecessary work-up of abnormalities that are extremely unlikely to cause harm. In my experience, this heuristic often affects the treatment of VIPs, where the fear of regret can be a particularly strong emotion.

Representativeness, availability, framing, anchoring, and regret have been shown repeatedly to affect judgment and decision making, even of highly trained professionals. Your awareness of these pitfalls will make you a better radiologist by helping you fight your natural human tendencies to make suboptimal decisions.

Using Theory to Answer Practical Questions

Any great theory should help us make sense of life's pragmatic questions, rather than simply beckon us to admire its abstract beauty. We will now review how decision theory can help us analyze a few nagging questions that arise in the daily practice of radiology.

The Toss-up

In the 1980s, Drs. Jerome Kassirer and Stephen Pauker established a unique consultation service at Tufts New England Medical Center, which prepared formal decision models (like the one in Figure 74) to advise referring clinicians on the best course of action for patients who posed diagnostic and therapeutic dilemmas.[271] As a result of their experience, they published what still remains one of my favorite editorials. Entitled "The Toss-up," it dealt with a recurring clinical dilemma: "Considerable turmoil is often created when expert physicians have different and strongly held opinions about the optimal treatment strategy for a given patient."[286]

Through decision analysis, Kassirer and Pauker found that these toss-ups, or close calls, often represented decisions in which "the consequences of divergent choices are, on the average, virtually identical." In other words, when the debate is most heated, the likely reason is because it doesn't matter. This beautiful insight has the potential to reduce the amount of hot air in radiology reading rooms everywhere.

The Value of a Negative Study

In the privacy of the reading room, radiologists sometimes denigrate referring clinicians who order tests that almost always yield normal results. These clinicians seem to be wasting our time. Why would someone order a test with such a low probability of finding significant disease? The answer lies in the significant harm that can be caused by many diseases if undiagnosed. Therefore, a referring clinician with impeccable judgment might logically order a test with a low yield to avoid missing a serious disease. (Screening mammography is a good example.) Decision theory reminds us that not all low probability imaging scenarios are created equal.[46]

Belief Update or Posterior Probability?

One implicit controversy—not discussed much, but ever-present—concerns the information the radiology report should provide. Are the words in the report intended to convey the post-test probability of disease to the referring clinician? Or should the report narrative tell the referring clinician how he or she should update the pre-test probability of disease? As we discussed in Chapter 10, these are two completely different concepts: The latter is an update to our belief, analogous to the likelihood ratio; the former is the belief itself, after taking into account the imaging evidence.

How we resolve this dilemma depends on who knows more about the patient. In other words, what is the relative weight of imaging evidence relative to the nonimaging information available from symptoms, physical exam, and other diagnostic tests? The degree of narrowing in the renal artery tells us almost everything we need to know to calculate the post-test probability of a hemodynamically significant stenosis. So we can provide a post-test probability of disease.

On the other hand, air-space opacities at the lung bases may represent atelectasis or pneumonia, depending on many other clinical factors. Thus, the best approach when interpreting such a chest radiograph is to convey how the imaging findings might update a referring clinician's belief, rather than to make a definitive conclusion in the report.

Foundation for a Lifetime

Every month, scientific journals publish an avalanche of new diagnostic imaging knowledge. Radiologists, like all physicians, must be lifelong learners. The essential tools reviewed in Chapters 10 and 11, such as sensitivity, specificity, and decision theory, can help radiologists interpret research results, and apply them in clinical practice. They also provide a firm foundation for the diagnostic reasoning we communicate in our radiology reports.

Part III:
The Future

Chapter 12:
The Future of Radiology Reporting

> *It's tough to make predictions, especially about the future.*
> —*Yogi Berra*

Radiology 2025

Intense and accelerating change will likely affect health care in the years ahead. Health care reimbursement, health care delivery, and therefore the practice of radiology will be radically different in 10 years.[287] Inevitably, provider payments will be based more heavily on the health of their patient population, not the number of patients seen or the number of procedures performed. What follows is an admittedly utopian vision of what health care might look like in 2025, intended to illustrate some of the forces likely to shape the future of the radiology report.

The Primary Care Encounter

In the future, physicians and patients will have no incentives for "patient visits." Whenever possible, patients will interact with their health care providers via secure email, messaging apps, and real-time video. Because the referring clinician and the radiologist will have an incentive to do the correct test and only the correct test, evidence-based clinical decision support will be universally available at the time of the imaging request, based on a standard exam code and a clearly specified reason for the study.[288,289] Smart phone apps will be used to schedule imaging studies, generate automated reminders for appropriate test preparation, directions to the imaging facility, and other study-specific information the patient may need.

Patient Arrival

Because health insurance companies will pay for value, not volume, no administrative barriers, such as "pre-certification" and other forms of utilization management, will be designed to reduce study volume.[290] Once a study is scheduled, the radiology practice, the primary care provider, and the payer will work together to ensure the patient undergoes the correct study without delay. The patient will be unaware of this behind-the-scenes work, which will be as seamless as the background work between online stores, credit card companies, and shipping companies to ensure a purchased item arrives on time at your doorstep.

By the time the patient arrives in the radiology suite, the radiology practice will have already identified the device, the protocol, and the technologist who will perform the exam. After identity verification, the patient will be escorted immediately to the imaging area.

Creation of Images

Because radiology systems will be embedded in the electronic medical record (EMR), the patient's complete clinical history will be immediately available to radiologists and technologists, including the documentation describing the referring clinician's thinking at the time the study was ordered. The EMR information will be summarized automatically in a single screen that displays data relevant to the upcoming imaging study. The technologist and radiologist will collaborate in advance to select the optimal imaging protocol for the patient.[291] Because a standard nomenclature for imaging protocols will be available on every imaging device, the desired protocol will be preselected on the imaging console when the patient is identified from the work list.

The acquired images will be sent to an advanced imaging laboratory, where initial image processing is performed automatically, triggered by the exam code and the protocol. If necessary, a specially trained technologist will perform additional post-processing, including measurements and annotations.

Image Interpretation and Reporting

The PACS (picture archiving and communication system) will automatically display the images in the correct configuration based on the exam code, imaging protocol, and reason for the exam. The radiology practice will agree on a default report template for each study, which will be selected automatically based on the exam code and reason for the study. Protocol steps and measurements from the advanced imaging laboratory will be prefilled into designated fields in the template.[292] The radiologist will briefly review and confirm the prefilled draft radiology report. The radiologist will devote nearly every minute to reviewing the images rather than reporting. Additional diagnostic information will be entered by means of trigger words, templates, or brief narrative dictation. Speech recognition accuracy will approach 100% by capitalizing on information about grammar and semantics.[293] Speech recognition systems will automatically suggest alternatives when a word is in doubt, similar to type-ahead on your smart phone.

When the report is complete, the radiologist will assign a global assessment code to the report, similar to a BI-RADS® (Breast Imaging Reporting and Data System) code, to indicate the level of risk that the imaging findings pose to the patient.[62] Any follow-up recommendations will clearly indicate the imaging modality and the time interval. Reporting tools will facilitate insertion of hyperlinks to key images directly from the narrative, creating a multimedia report.[153] Standard exam codes[231] will ensure radiation exposure data and other key performance indicators are benchmarked by national registries.[232]

Automated Radiologist Assistance

The reporting system will serve as an intelligent agent that assists in creating a high-quality report.[234] The system will detect reporting errors in real-time, such as gender mismatches and left-right inconsistencies.[294] Before finalization, the system will remind the radiologist to include essential elements of the report based on expert guidelines, including appropriate follow-up for incidental findings, such as adrenal or lung nodules. Natural language processing will extract data from the narrative portion of the report to populate the patient's EMR.[295–297] Data from the report will trigger relevant decision support for the radiologist, such as a related teaching case, a relevant consensus guideline, a similar radiology report, or a gamut for the imaging findings.[298] Probabilistic reasoning systems will suggest differential diagnostic considerations.[299–302]

Communication of Results

Global assessment codes will communicate actionable report information, which is highlighted in the EMR, much like an abnormal laboratory value. Any urgent information will be transmitted automatically to the clinical team through nonroutine channels, such as smart phones. The care team will acknowledge each recommendation, indicating whether they intend to follow it.[62] Health care facilities will maintain accurate information about the care team for each patient. If the clinical team has any questions, the radiologist will be available to answer questions in one click, including by means of a phone call, secure text message, electronic mail, and screen sharing. Non-urgent actionable assessment codes will be monitored electronically to close the loop. Systems will send timed reminders, ensuring that patients receive recommended follow-up.

Performance Improvement

A comprehensive program to monitor and improve radiologist diagnostic performance will analyze the outcome of each global assessment code. The usage rate and outcome of each code will be tracked for each radiologist, much like the BI-RADS usage of breast imagers can be tracked today.[222,303] Variability among radiologists will be analyzed to find exemplary radiologists to emulate and others who may need additional training.

Image Exchange

After a short delay during which referring clinicians review the report, patients will have full access to their reports and images over the Internet through secure patient portals. Universal cloud-based image exchange will eliminate the need for CDs, DVDs, and other portable media to transmit images among providers.[304]

The Radiology 2025 Vision

This vision of the future of radiology patient care anticipates a well-designed, collaborative process requiring each member of the team to operate at the "top of their license," leaving the team both challenged and fulfilled. We now move on to imagine the future of the radiology report in more detail.

The Radiology Report in 2025

Consistency is a hallmark of quality. What draws us to the burgers at Five Guys or the desserts at the Cheesecake Factory is the consistency of the product across time and location. Such consistency will be the watchword for the radiology report in 2025. Reports dictated by Dr. Jones will be organized the same on Monday as on Friday. And Dr. Smith's reports on Tuesday will be organized the same as Dr. Jones' reports on Monday.

Although regulatory imperatives and certification requirements will force some standardization, the strongest drivers of structured radiology reporting will be referring clinicians, who have precious little time to spend reading radiology reports and who prefer a consistently organized report.

These radiology reports will be asked to serve multiple purposes. They will be transmitted to clinical systems to become a part of the patient's legal medical record. But they also will be viewed by referring clinicians on smart phones and tablets. And they will be viewed by patients in online personal health records. Finally, reports will be reused for data mining and analytics to answer questions of quality, productivity, and safety. For example, radiology practices want to know: How many reports dictated by trainees overnight are modified by attending radiologists in the morning? How compliant is our practice with the documentation requirements for critical result communication? How many reports contained left/right or male/female errors? These are difficult questions to answer without some standardization to aid in extracting, filtering, and quantifying information from radiology reports.

The Future of Speech Recognition

Despite the significant progress in speech recognition accuracy over the past 2 decades, the technology is still in its adolescence. One likely area of rapid change is the intersection of speech recognition and mobile devices. The capabilities that enable the cell phone to respond to our spoken commands could just as easily perform cloud-based speech recognition or control a radiology reporting system. Already today, some systems include verbal commands to jump to a specific field, fill in a field with a phrase triggered by a key word, or execute a command, such as "sign off report."

Another promising opportunity for improvement is the use of context and semantics to improve speech recognition accuracy. Cloud-based speech recognition systems can now aggregate very large databases of matched sound and text, to which machine learning techniques can be applied to improve performance. Many of the crazy errors made by speech recognition systems, such as "the Super Bowl of the right kidney," would never occur if the computer knew of the meaning of those words. Likewise, knowledge of context, such as the modality used and body region being reviewed, can enhance speech recognition. For example, word frequencies, and the tri-gram algorithms on which speech recognition is based, change dramatically based on the exam code.[293]

Word frequency varies widely among the sections of the report. The word "cancer" is much less likely to appear in the Technique section than in the body of the report or in the Clinical History section. The reverse is true of phrases such as "3 Tesla magnet." As these improvements take hold, speech recognition systems will approach true natural language understanding— electronically extracting discrete semantic information from narrative text using machine learning.

Continued progress in this area is inevitable, but technology will never provide a "free lunch" for radiologists, enabling them to dictate as they please and expecting computers to come along afterward to understand and codify what they meant. As a result, radiologists still will be expected to constrain their reporting habits, so computers can later extract some of the meaning from radiology reports.

Attribute-Value Format

Standardization of radiologists' reports will appear first in the Observations section. For those reports with a repetitive set of organs that need to be reviewed, such as the lungs, heart, and tubes and lines in an ICU chest study, or the liver, pancreas, and kidneys in an abdominal CT study, an *attribute-value* construction will facilitate rapid processing of information by the report reader.[24,40,41]

Compare this:

```
The lungs are clear.  The heart is normal in
size.
```

To this:

```
Lungs: Clear

Heart: Normal in size
```

Prefilling the Radiology Report

Radiologists often spend time dictating information that is already available elsewhere. For example, the technologist already specifies each MR and CT protocol step before it is performed. Why should the radiologist redictate this information? Several reporting systems now can be configured to receive and automatically prefill report fields with information from other sources—thereby increasing the accuracy and efficiency of the radiologist.[292] This capability will expand in the years to come.

Imagine the possibilities: Computer-based provider order entry (CPOE) systems capture clinical history in electronic form, which could be transmitted electronically to the reporting system. Measurements and other image annotations created by technologists in an advanced imaging laboratory, or by the radiologist in the reading room, also could be pulled into reports directly. Intelligent contrast agent injectors track the amount and rate of contrast material administered. Automatic transmission of these data to the radiology report would be a refreshing change from the game of "telephone" that requires the technologist to remember and jot down the contrast agent specifics in a place where the radiologist can view and redictate them. Recent legislation makes radiation dose tracking a similar imperative. In many states, practices are finding ways to prefill dose information in the radiology report.

These many forms of pre-filled of report information will foster enhanced clinical documentation and better revenue capture.

Global Assessments

Most radiology work lists prioritize urgent exams to the top of the list. But when I dictate two reports, one containing a life-threatening critical test result and the other a normal result on a healthy outpatient, they look identical on the referring clinician's list of test results to review in the EMR.

In the future, an abnormal radiology result will be identified and highlighted in the EMR just like an abnormal serum potassium value. Global assessment codes will be assigned to most reports. Likewise, standard methods for documenting recommendations will ensure that appropriate follow-up tests are performed as recommended. For certain recurring exams, such as ICU chest exams, global assessments may denote improvement, worsening, or no change of chronic findings.

Structured Report Databases

Because perfectly accurate natural language processing techniques are unlikely to be achieved, the radiologist occasionally will need to select specific report elements from a predefined list. For example, a practice might decide to capture a consistent measure of the severity of pancreatitis or the malignant potential of a liver lesion. In collaboration with referring clinicians, radiology practices will identify the essential reporting needs of a few select clinical situations. These documentation requirements can seriously affect radiologist productivity if not implemented properly, and thus should be considered carefully. But in the right circumstances, they will provide substantial clinical value—for example, tracking the standardized uptake values of oncology lesions to plot disease progression over time.

As more radiology report information is discretely documented, analytic tools will measure, and thereby improve, the performance of radiologists. Radiologists interpreting chest radiography will know how their chest CT recommendation rate compares with that of their colleagues. And they will know how often the recommended chest CT studies capture clinically significant disease. As the BI-RADS experience has shown, tracking these proxies for radiologist accuracy measurement provides constructive feedback to individual radiologists for continuous improvement.[176]

As structured information is captured in real-time, a new realm of decision support will become available to the radiologist. Automated reasoning methods that have been available to other specialties for years[305] will provide radiologists with recommendations for lesion follow-up or diagnostic suggestions for unusual cases.[234] Likewise, structured report information could trigger automatic retrieval of online teaching files or peer-reviewed literature relevant to specific clinical cases. This new information could supplant other retrospective sources of clinical research data, such as administrative claims, which have substantial limitations for use in diagnostic imaging research.[306]

More Sophisticated Radiology Report Templates

A recently approved a new radiology template standard[205] will make report information accessible to many other software applications, such as result communication systems, EMR systems, decision support systems, and analytic systems. As vendors adopt this new standard, template fields will contain not just text, but also menus, numbers, dates, and times, making standard responses and range checking possible. Fields in these new templates will accept data from other sources, such as the EMR, the radiology information system (RIS), or the imaging modality. Some practices already use a similar feature to prefill measurements made on vascular and pregnancy ultrasound studies into the appropriate fields for the radiologist to review. This transfer avoids the tedium and mistakes that can occur from repetitively redictating that information. Steve Horii at the University of Pennsylvania found that this feature yielded an approximately 40% reduction in the time to produce first-trimester ultrasound reports and a 30% reduction in the time to produce second-trimester reports. This bears repeating: a structured reporting feature that saves radiologists time!

The new template standard will give practice leaders new tools to manage radiology reporting behavior in their practices. Each field has one of three behaviors when the report is finalized: (a) The field can be silent, which is the only behavior that most reporting vendors currently provide; (b) it can be marked to alert the radiologist when it has not been modified; or (c) it can be marked to prohibit finalization of the report until the field is modified.

These new features and others will be available for any compliant template library, including one created by a reporting vendor, your radiology practice, or another professional group.

Tip: Urge your reporting vendor to develop authoring and editing tools that make these more sophisticated templates easy to create.

The Multimedia Report

We live in a world filled with billions of web pages, each a multimedia mixture of images, text, and even videos—much more engaging than the bland unformatted text that comprises most radiology reports. It's puzzling that an image-based specialty like radiology doesn't make multimedia radiology reports just as commonplace.[147,152,153] A key image is worth a thousand-word report. Many patients and referring clinicians appreciate seeing first-hand the best picture of the pathology, as identified by the radiologist.[153]

But multimedia radiology reports haven't taken hold for one simple reason. Health care information technology is woefully behind the times. RISs, which store and transmit radiology reports, are often based on decades-old technology. And electronic interfaces that transmit information between the RIS and EMRs use messaging standards, such as Health Level 7 (HL7), that are decades old and cannot easily accommodate text formatting, let alone images.

Unlike the Internet, where text and images grew up together, early systems for managing medical images required blistering transmission speeds and more robust computational power—magnitudes greater than the speeds needed for managing text reports. Consequently, the two infrastructures grew up separately, and our early adoption of digital imaging technology led to a paradoxic schism between the worlds of medical records and medical images. Even today, a clinical image formatted according to JPEG, the most common format for Internet images, is easy to transmit and display in a web browser. But this format does not support image operations that are essential for clinical interpretation, such as adjustment of window and level.

New standards are emerging to integrate clinical images and web technologies. Web access to DICOM objects (DICOMweb), HL7 clinical document architecture (HL7 CDA), and Fast Healthcare Interoperability Resources (FHIR) are reaching the adoption tipping point, enabling truly integrated systems for transmitting images and reports and motivating radiology vendors to provide efficient platforms for creating multimedia reports. Another reinforcing trend is the accelerating adoption of RIS modules embedded in the EMR, which will obviate transmission interfaces altogether. These integrated systems, based on modern standards, will be designed from the ground up to support all aspects of a radiologist's work, including the ability to create multimedia reports efficiently.[307] The integration of images and reports will be a long-awaited and revolutionary change.

Natural Language Processing

The latest natural language processing (NLP) techniques, which automatically dissect even the meatiest clinical prose into small digital morsels, provide another early look at how information technology will shape the future of radiology reporting. For example, the Lexicon Mediated Entropy Reduction (LEXIMER) system can classify reports as either positive or negative and can detect reports that contain clinical recommendations.[295] Other systems have attempted to extract all clinically useful concepts from reports, not just a few key attributes. For example, the Medical Language Extraction and Encoding System (MEDLEE), developed over 20 years at Columbia-Presbyterian Medical Center, parsed the text of radiology reports into a structured database by using a locally created vocabulary.[308,309] MEDLEE has been evaluated for 24 clinical conditions based on 150 manually labeled radiology reports.[178,296]

These systems can extract concepts with an accuracy comparable to that of human experts under controlled conditions. The Columbia team has already published examples of the beneficial use of MEDLEE in specific limited clinical settings.[310] The underlying rule-based annotation tools are not easily scalable because of the time and experimentation needed to account for the ambiguous and inconsistent use of language in radiology reports.[311] And MEDLEE did face challenges when it was applied across institutions,[312] or to more complex reports from cross-sectional imaging.[313] But it demonstrated the potential value of NLP in radiology.

Several vendors now sell systems that detect reports with specific characteristics, such as billing and quality errors (see Figure 75).

	Critical values
Quality characteristics	Male/female discrepancies
	Left/right discrepancies
	Contrast exams dictated with no mention of IV contrast in the report
Billing characteristics	Complete abdominal ultrasound with no mentioned of key organs
	Discrepancy between billing code and number of views in the report

Figure 75. Report features detected by natural language processing (NLP) in current vendor products.

Machine Learning

Machine learning addresses the intractability of manually building rules to extract and classify specific clinical concepts from clinical narrative. Rather than a laborious manual tuning process, the machine itself analyzes large databases of reports and automatically learns from the data to construct more general concept extraction algorithms. Several machine learning NLP systems have focused on radiology reports and other clinical documents.[314] As these algorithms become more accurate over time, they will enable even more sophisticated technologies, such as report similarity measures, automated summarization, and the conversion of reports into lay language.

NLP will play a vital role in the analysis of the massive historical record of narrative reports. For example, based on the model of imaging observations described in Chapter 2, my laboratory has developed a machine-learning system to extract key concepts from narrative reports.[315] But NLP techniques, like radiology interpretation itself, are never perfectly accurate, especially when no attempt has been made to standardize report content. In the future, standardized reporting at the time of report creation will be paired with NLP techniques to extract vital information from the accompanying narrative. Structured reporting and NLP, working together, will have synergistic effects on our ability to reuse information from the radiology report.

The Future of Report Communication

The single biggest problem in communication is the illusion that it has taken place.
—*George Bernard Shaw*

Nonroutine Communication

Sometimes, the report is not enough. In emergent or other nonroutine clinical situations, the interpreting physician must expedite the delivery of a diagnostic imaging report (preliminary or final) in a manner that reasonably ensures timely receipt of the findings.

The American College of Radiology's (ACR's) Practice Parameter for Communication of Diagnostic Imaging Findings[131] outlines three scenarios in which nonroutine communication is warranted.

Findings that suggest a need for immediate or urgent intervention, such as pneumothorax, pneumoperitoneum, or a significantly misplaced line or tube,

Findings that are discrepant with a preceding interpretation of the same examination and for which failure to act may adversely affect patient health, and

Findings that the interpreting physician reasonably believes may be seriously adverse to the patient's health and are unexpected by the treating or referring physician.

Several vendors now offer phone-based closed-loop communication systems for these urgent, discrepant, and adverse unexpected findings, which ensure that 100% of results have documented communication. And we are already seeing analogies to social media communication, including companies that offer smart phone notifications via secure text messages and those that offer a private Facebook-like page for each patient, including a "newsfeed" of test results and other communications.

All of these technologies ensure that there is a record of the person notified and the date and time of the communication, a requirement of the Joint Commission[103] and the ACR. From the ACR policy:

Interpreting physicians should document all non-routine communications and include the time and method of communication and specifically name the person to whom the communication was delivered. Documentation is best placed in the radiology report or the patient's medical record.

In addition, many hospital policies require that critical results be communicated in-person or over the phone, with read-back required for confirmation.

Test results are typically stratified into three categories: red (critical), orange, and yellow. Figure 76 below shows a stratification recently endorsed by the ACR.[316] A similar system is used by the Brigham and Women's Hospital.[317]

Priority	Description	Example	Communication
Red (critical)	Potentially immediately life threatening	Tension pneumothorax, intestinal ischemia, intracranial hemorrhage	Within minutes
Orange	Possible mortality or significant morbidity within 2 or 3 days	Intra-abdominal abscess, bone at risk for pathologic fracture	Within hours
Yellow	Possible mortality or significant morbidity, but not urgent	Lung nodule not clearly benign, hemodynamically significant stenosis	Within days

Figure 76. Color-coded priorities for radiology test results.[316,317]

The Future of Electronic Access by Patients

Two trends are combining to accelerate patients' online access to their own medical records: meaningful use incentives, which include a goal to make test results available to patients, and the wide availability of vendor products that enable online patient engagement. My previous employer ran an advertising campaign for their patient portal using the tag line, "Finally, get your medical records like you get your music."

Direct communication with patients is routine in mammography, for which sending a letter to the patient summarizing her results is mandated by federal law. And providing reports directly to patients is nothing new: Most patients can obtain their reports on paper or CD as soon as they are available, often in a matter of hours, simply by requesting them from the "film library" (or whatever it may be called it in this post-film world). But the convenience and proactive nature of patient portals make them a compelling trend.

The release of reports can be controversial for some referring clinicians, who worry about an avalanche of patient questions about report content or the danger of patients receiving bad news without a compassionate caregiver to consult. Other referring clinicians are concerned that patients might contact the radiologist, who has only a partial picture of the patient and may be unaware of competing health problems and social and emotional factors that influence the patient's perceptions of test results.

My former and my current institution now release reports to patients (after a delay that enables referring clinicians to prevent release if they wish). Despite these systems, the rate of direct contact between patient and radiologist remains extremely low, and there has been no appreciable effect on patient phone calls to referring clinician practices. Our experience is consistent with the data from other organizations: The patients love it.[318] In time, we will see technologies designed to enhance how patients experience their radiology reports—systems that tailor the report language for patients' reading level or that provide hyperlinks to layman's definitions of clinical terms.

Patient Expectations for Radiology Reports

As patients gain ready access to their reports online, radiologists will be held to their higher expectations. Consider the abdominal CT study of a patient who has undergone a cholecystectomy. The radiologist might forget to alter a standard template that states that "the gallbladder is normal." A referring clinician might understand that mistake as a minor clerical error. On the other hand, a patient encountering such an erroneous report may draw the conclusion that the radiologist reviewed the wrong patient's images.

Release of radiology reports is only one of many attractive patient portal functions, such as the ability to request or cancel clinic appointments or to review lab results, allergies, medications, and problem lists. Regardless of the challenges of electronic access by patients, its growing prevalence will require radiology practices to adapt.

The Possible Extinction of the Radiology Report

If you dislike change, you're going to dislike irrelevance even
more.
—Eric Shinseki

Very little has changed about radiology reporting since the first reports were first produced over a century ago. Consider the letter shown in Figure 77, written by Dr. Morton to his referring clinician colleague shortly after he penned the report we examined in Chapter 1.

```
Dear Doctor Stieglitz,

In regard to the proper charges to make to your pa-
tient, I find it difficult to decide and I am most
willing to be guided to a great extent by you.

My usual charge to radiograph through the entire body
is $100.  But like all physicians' services a negative
result is harder to charge for than an affirmative one.
If we had found the stone in the kidney it would have
been worth that money, but we didn't.  I think there-
fore it will be fair to say $75.
```

Figure 77. A letter illustrating that the radiology fee-for-service model has a long history. (Reproduced with permission from the New York Academy of Medicine Library.)

Even our financial model remains the same as a century ago. But the drivers of change are powerful and difficult to ignore. New health care payment models, which no longer pay per study, are already being tried in many areas. Since the radiology report is the primary artifact that justifies payment for our work, its very existence may be called into question. In the end, perhaps "the radiology report" as we know it will become extinct.

Imagine a world in which a full radiology report was produced only if it contributed clinically relevant information. For many absolutely normal studies, do we need to produce a report at all? When a chest radiographic study from the ICU is interpreted, is it sufficient in most cases to indicate whether the chronic findings are better or worse? Perhaps the information in a radiology report should be delivered piecemeal, or not at all, based on priority. Once the financial straitjacket of "one study, one report" is removed, innovators will capitalize on the opportunity to establish more efficient models of radiology communication.

This transformation will certainly involve "interesting times." But if radiologists welcome these advances in the use of words, sentences, and paragraphs in the same way they have already embraced the innovative display of pixels, voxels, and images, radiologists and the reports they create will emerge even stronger, ready for the next wave of innovation.

References

1.   The X-Ray in Medicine; Some Experiments Made before Doctors of This City. *New York Times* (1896). at <http://timesmachine.nytimes.com/timesmachine/1896/04/28/108 229569.html?pageNumber=1>

2.   Morton, W. J. & Hammer, E. W. *The X-Ray or Photography of the Invisible and Its Value in Surgery.* (American Technical Book Company, 1896).

3.   Reiner, BI, Knight, N. Reinventing the Radiology Report: Part I, A History. *AXIS Imaging* (2004). at <http://www.axisimagingnews.com/2004/11/reinventing-the-radiology-report-part-i-a-history/>

4.   Grigg, E. *The Trail of the Invisible Light: From X-Strahlen to Radio (Bio) logy.* (Charles C. Thomas, 1965).

5.   Hickey, P. Standardization of Roentgen Ray Reports. *Am. J. Roentgenol.* 422–425 (1922). at <http://books.google.com/books?id=XFZGAAAAYAAJ>

6.   Sistrom, C., Lanier, L. & Mancuso, A. Reporting Instruction for Radiology Residents. *Acad. Radiol.* **11,** 76–84 (2004).

7.   Williamson, K. B. *et al.* Assessing Radiology Resident Reporting Skills. *Radiology* **225,** 719–722 (2002).

8. Landro, L. Radiologists Push for Medical Reports Patients Can Understand. *Wall Street Journal* (2014). at <http://www.wsj.com/articles/radiologists-push-for-medical-reports-patients-can-understand-1410724814>

9. Coakley, F. V *et al.* Routine Editing of Trainee-Generated Radiology Reports: Effect on Style Quality. *Acad. Radiol.* **10,** 289–294 (2003).

10. Collard, M. D., Tellier, J., Chowdhury, A. S. M. I. & Lowe, L. H. Improvement in Reporting Skills of Radiology Residents with a Structured Reporting Curriculum. *Acad. Radiol.* **21,** 126–133 (2014).

11. Coakley, F. V., Liberman, L. & Panicek, D. M. Style Guidelines for Radiology Reporting: A Manner of Speaking. *Am. J. Roentgenol.* **180,** 327–328 (2003).

12. Ridley, L. J. Guide to the Radiology Report. *Australas. Radiol.* **46,** 366–369 (2002).

13. Wallis, A. & McCoubrie, P. The Radiology Report--Are We Getting the Message Across? *Clin. Radiol.* **66,** 1015–1022 (2011).

14. Hall, F. M. Language of the Radiology Report Primer for Residents and Wayward Radiologists. *Am. J. Roentgenol.* **175,** 1239–1242 (2000).

15. Paris, A. *Handbook of Radiologic Dictation.* (ProScan MRI Education Foundation, 2004).

16. Pool, F. & Goergen, S. Quality of the Written Radiology Report: A Review of the Literature. *J. Am. Coll. Radiol.* **7,** 634–643 (2010).

17. Steele, J. L., Nyce, J. M., Williamson, K. B. & Gunderman, R. B. Learning to Report. *Acad. Radiol.* **9,** 817–820 (2002).

18. Gunn, A. J. *et al.* Structured Feedback from Referring Physicians: A Novel Approach to Quality Improvement in Radiology Reporting. *AJR. Am. J. Roentgenol.* **201,** 853–857 (2013).

19. Sobel, J. L. *et al.* Information Content and Clarity Of Radiologists' Reports for Chest Radiography. *Acad. Radiol.* **3,** 709–717 (1996).

20. Clinger, N. J., Hunter, T. B. & Hillman, B. J. Radiology Reporting: Attitudes of Referring Physicians. *Radiology* **169,** 825–826 (1988).

21. Lafortune, M., Breton, G. & Baudouin, J. L. The Radiological Report: What Is Useful for the Referring Physician? *Can. Assoc. Radiol. J.* **39,** 140–143 (1988).

22. McLoughlin, R. F., So, C. B., Gray, R. R. & Brandt, R. Radiology Reports: How Much Descriptive Detail Is Enough? *Am. J. Roentgenol.* **165,** 803–806 (1995).

23. Gagliardi, R. A. The Evolution of the X-ray Report. *AJR. Am. J. Roentgenol.* **164,** 501–502 (1995).

24. Naik, S. S., Hanbidge, A. & Wilson, S. R. Radiology Reports: Examining Radiologist and Clinician Preferences Regarding Style and Content. *Am. J. Roentgenol.* **176,** 591–598 (2001).

25. Heilman, R. S. What's Wrong with Radiology. *N. Engl. J. Med.* **306,** 477–479 (1982).

26. Manzone, T. A., Malkowicz, S. B., Tomaszewski, J. E., Schnall, M. D. & Langlotz, C. P. Use of Endorectal MR Imaging to Predict Prostate Carcinoma Recurrence after Radical Prostatectomy. *Radiology* **209,** 537–542 (1998).

27. Carroll, L. *Through the Looking-Glass, and What Alice Found There.* (1871).

28. Osler, W. On the Educational Value of the Medical Society. *Bost. Med Surg J* **148,** 275–279 (1903).

29. Sierra, A. E., Bisesi, M. A., Rosenbaum, T. L. & Potchen, E. J. Readability of the Radiologic Report. *Invest. Radiol.* **27,** 236–239 (1992).

30. Friedman, P. J. Radiologic Reporting: Structure. *Am. J. Roentgenol.* **140,** 171–172 (1983).

31. Friedman, P. J. Radiologic Reporting: the Hierarchy of Terms. *Am. J. Roentgenol.* **140,** 402–403 (1983).

32. Ly, J. Q. The Rigler Sign. *Radiology* **228,** 706–707 (2003).

33. Koga, T. & Fujimoto, K. Images in Clinical Medicine. Kerley's A, B, and C lines. *N. Engl. J. Med.* **360,** 1539 (2009).

34. Vick, C. W. Unremarkable Words Redux. *J. Am. Coll. Radiol.* **9,** 453–4 (2012).

35.   Safire, W. *Lend Me Your Ears: Great Speeches In History*. (W. W. Norton and Company, 2004).

36.   Lee, R., Cohen, M. D. & Jennings, G. S. A New Method of Evaluating the Quality of Radiology Reports. *Acad. Radiol.* **13,** 241–248 (2006).

37.   Penn, W. *Fruits of Solitude, in Reflections and Maxims Relating to the Conduct of Human Life*. (Benjamin Johnson, 1792).

38.   Berlin, L. Radiology Reports. *AJR. Am. J. Roentgenol.* **169,** 943–946 (2013).

39.   Gawande, A. *The Checklist Manifesto: How to Get Things Right*. (Henry Holt and Company, 2009).

40.   Schwartz, L. H., Panicek, D. M., Berk, A. R., Li, Y. & Hricak, H. Improving Communication of Diagnostic Radiology Findings through Structured Reporting. *Radiology* **260,** 174–181 (2011).

41.   Manoonchai, N. *et al.* Satisfaction of Imaging Report Rendered in Emergency Setting: A Survey of Radiology and Referring Physicians. *Acad. Radiol.* **22,** 760–770 (2015).

42.   Bosmans, J. M. L., Weyler, J. J., De Schepper, A. M. & Parizel, P. M. The Radiology Report as Seen by Radiologists and Referring Clinicians: Results of the COVER and ROVER Surveys. *Radiology* **259,** 184 –195 (2011).

43.   Vick, C. W. Lexicon for Uncertain Times. *J. Am. Coll. Radiol.* **7,** 827–828 (2010).

44.   Enfield, C. The Scope of the Roentgenologist's Report. *JAMA J. Am. Med. Assoc.* **80,** 999–1001 (1923).

45.   Plumb, A. A. O., Grieve, F. M. & Khan, S. H. Survey of Hospital Clinicians' Preferences Regarding the Format of Radiology Reports. *Clin. Radiol.* **64,** 386–396 (2009).

46.   Gorry, G. A., Pauker, S. G. & Schwartz, W. B. The Diagnostic Importance of the Normal Finding. *N. Engl. J. Med.* **298,** 486–489 (1978).

47.   Jefferson, T. Letter from Thomas Jefferson to Thomas Jefferson Randolph. *Founders Online National Archive* at <http://founders.archives.gov/documents/Jefferson/99-01-02-9249>

48. Singh, H., Spitzmueller, C., Petersen, N. I. O. and M. T. R. in E. H. R.-B. S., Sawhney, M. K. & Sittig, D. F. Information Overload and Missed Test Results in Electronic Health Record-Based Settings. *JAMA Intern. Med.* **173,** 702–4 (2013).

49. Ginsberg, L. E. 'If Clinically Indicated:' Is It? *Radiology* **254,** 324–325 (2010).

50. Waley, A. in *The Analects of Confucius 2:17* (Knopf, 2000).

51. Khorasani, R. *et al.* Is Terminology Used Effectively to Convey Diagnostic Certainty in Radiology Reports? *Acad. Radiol.* **10,** 685–8 (2003).

52. Hobby, J. L., Tom, B. D., Todd, C., Bearcroft, P. W. & Dixon, A. K. Communication of Doubt and Certainty in Radiological Reports. *Br. J. Radiol.* **73,** 999–1001 (2000).

53. Kong, A., Barnett, G. O., Mosteller, F. & Youtz, C. How Medical Professionals Evaluate Expressions of Probability. *N. Engl. J. Med.* **315,** 740–744 (1986).

54. Berlin, L. Pitfalls of the Vague Radiology Report. *AJR. Am. J. Roentgenol.* **174,** 1511–1518 (2000).

55. Chesbrough, R. Malpractice Monitor: Vagueness in Report Can Work against You. *Diagnostic Imaging* (2003). at <http://www.diagnosticimaging.com/dimag/legacy/db_area/archives/2003/0312.malpractice.di.shtml>

56. Bosmans, J. M. L., Peremans, L., De Schepper, A. M., Duyck, P. O. & Parizel, P. M. How Do Referring Clinicians Want Radiologists to Report? Suggestions from the COVER Survey. *Insights Imaging* **2,** 577–584 (2011).

57. Orel, S. G., Kay, N., Reynolds, C. & Sullivan, D. C. BI-RADS Categorization as a Predictor of Malignancy. *Radiology* **211,** 845–850 (1999).

58. Keats, TE, Sistrom, C. *Atlas of Radiologic Measurement.* (Mosby, 2001).

59. Kelvin, Lord. in *Popular Lectures and Addresses* (1872).

60. Hall, F. M. 'Mild' and 'Slight.' *Am. J. Roentgenol.* **169,** 315 (1997).

61. Kijowski, R., Blankenbaker, D., Stanton, P., Fine, J. & De Smet, A. Arthroscopic Validation of Radiographic Grading Scales of Osteoarthritis of the Tibiofemoral Joint. *AJR. Am. J. Roentgenol.* **187,** 794–9 (2006).

62. Zafar, H. M. *et al.* Code Abdomen: An Assessment Coding Scheme for Abdominal Imaging Findings Possibly Representing Cancer. *J. Am. Coll. Radiol.* **12,** 947–950 (2015).

63. Ellison, R. *Invisible Man.* (Random House, 1995).

64. Hunter, T. B. Radiologic Reports: Structure and Review. *AJR. Am. J. Roentgenol.* **142,** 647–648 (1984).

65. Sistrom, C. L. *et al.* Recommendations for Additional Imaging in Radiology Reports: Multifactorial Analysis of 5.9 Million Examinations. *Radiology* **253,** 453–461 (2009).

66. Grieve, F. M., Plumb, A. A. & Khan, S. H. Radiology Reporting: A General Practitioner's Perspective. *Br. J. Radiol.* **83,** 17–22 (2010).

67. Baker, S. R. The Dictated Report and The Radiologist's Ethos. An Inextricable Relationship: Pitfalls to Avoid. *Eur. J. Radiol.* **83,** 236–238 (2014).

68. Hoang, J. K. Avoid 'Cannot Exclude': Make a Diagnosis. *J. Am. Coll. Radiol.* (2015). doi:10.1016/j.jacr.2015.06.018

69. Crews, F. *The Random House Handbook.* (McGraw-Hill, 1991).

70. Twain, M. Fenimore Cooper's Literary Offenses. (1895). at <http://twain.lib.virginia.edu/projects/rissetto/offense.html>

71. Strunk, W, White, E. *The Elements of Style.* (Longman, 1999).

72. Shehadi, W. More on Medical Terminology. *AJR. Am. J. Roentgenol.* **135,** 1118 (1980).

73. Pope, T. L. 'Conventional radiograph,' not 'plain film'. *Am. J. Roentgenol.* **170,** 1426 (1998).

74. Friedman, P. J. Radiologic Reporting: Describing the Lungs and Pleura. *AJR. Am. J. Roentgenol.* **140,** 1030–1031 (1983).

75. Trapnell, D. H. Radiologic Reporting. *Am. J. Roentgenol.* **142,** 233–234 (1984).

76. Tuddenham, W. J. In Defense of Opacity. *Radiographics* **6,** 171–172 (1986).

77. Rogers, L. F. What's in a Name? *Am. J. Roentgenol.* **170,** 1415 (1998).

78. Hall, F. M. & Movson, J. S. The Radiologic Hedge. *Am. J. Roentgenol.* **154,** 903–904 (1990).

79. Ronai, P. M. A Surfeit of Superfluous and Redundant Pleonasms. *AJR. Am. J. Roentgenol.* **160,** 412 (1993).

80. Berk, R. N. & Whalen, E. Impediments to Clarity: An Annotated Glossary of Rhetorical Pratfalls and Pitfalls. *AJR. Am. J. Roentgenol.* **159,** 1115–1121 (1992).

81. Bohrer, S. P. 'Nonspecific Gas Pattern'. *Radiology* **173,** 283 (1989).

82. Markus, J. B., Somers, S., Franic, S. E., Moola, C. & Stevenson, G. W. Interobserver Variation in the Interpretation of Abdominal Radiographs. *Radiology* **171,** 69–71 (1989).

83. Patel, N. H. & Lauber, P. R. The Meaning of a Nonspecific Abdominal Gas Pattern. *Acad. Radiol.* **2,** 667–669 (1995).

84. Hall, F. M. Medical Eponyms. *RadioGraphics* **26,** 1134 (2006).

85. Saint-Exupery, A. de. *Terre des Hommes.* (Le Livre de Poche, 1939).

86. Burke, E. *Letter to Richard Burke, Esq. on Protestant Ascendency in Ireland. The Works of the Right Honourable Edmund Burke* (1793). at <http://www.gutenberg.org/files/15702/15702-h/15702-h.htm#RICHARD_BURKE_ESQ>

87. Baker, S. R. & Partyka, L. Relative Importance of Metaphor in Radiology versus Other Medical Specialties. *Radiographics* **32,** 235–240 (2012).

88. Pinker, S. Communicating Science and Technology in the 21st Century. *MIT Video* (2012). at <http://mit.tv/U8pvhh>

89. Kumar, G., Kamath, V. & Murali, S. R. Nomenclature in the Journal of Hand Surgery. *J. Hand Surg. (British Eur. Vol.* **29,** 85–86 (2004).

90. Wraight, W. M., Smith, J. D. & Floyd, D. Nomenclature for Fingers and Phalanges: To Name or to Number? *J. Plast. Reconstr. Aesthetic Surg.* **60,** 368–371 (2007).

91.   Skillicorn, C. J. Do the Terms 'Proximal' and 'Distal' Cause Confusion Amongst Radiologists and Other Clinicians? *Clin. Radiol.* **64,** 397–402 (2009).

92.   Tuddenham, W. J. Editors Page: Of Antlers, Fish and Scrawny Children. *Radiographics* **3,** 545 (1983).

93.   Hall, F. M. Demise of Generic Terms 'Osteoporosis' and 'Osteopenia' in Radiology Reporting. *AJR. Am. J. Roentgenol.* **173,** 1127–1128 (1999).

94.   Lenchik, L., Rochmis, P. & Sartoris, D. J. Optimized Interpretation and Reporting of Dual X-ray Absorptiometry (DXA) Scans. *AJR. Am. J. Roentgenol.* **171,** 1509–1520 (1998).

95.   Kanis, J. A., Melton, L. J., Christiansen, C., Johnston, C. C. & Khaltaev, N. The Diagnosis of Osteoporosis. *J. Bone Miner. Res.* **9,** 1137–1141 (1994).

96.   Griscom, N. T. & Jaramillo, D. 'Osteoporosis,' 'Osteomalacia,' and 'Osteopenia': Proper Terminology in Childhood. *AJR. Am. J. Roentgenol.* **175,** 268–269 (2000).

97.   Patterson, H. S. & Sponaugle, D. N. Is Infiltrate a Useful Term in the Interpretation of Chest Radiographs? Physician Survey Results. *Radiology* **235,** 5–8 (2005).

98.   Hansell, D. M. *et al.* Fleischner Society: Glossary of Terms for Thoracic Imaging. *Radiology* **246,** 697–722 (2008).

99.   Wikipedia: Pronunciation Respelling Key. at <https://en.wikipedia.org/wiki/Wikipedia:Pronunciation_respelling_key>

100.   Wikipedia: Speech Recognition. at <https://en.wikipedia.org/wiki/Speech_recognition#Hidden_Markov_models>

101.   Ringler, M. D., Goss, B. C. & Bartholmai, B. J. Syntactic and Semantic Errors in Radiology Reports Associated with Speech Recognition Software. *Stud. Health Technol. Inform.* **216,** 922 (2015).

102.   Bhan, S. N., Coblentz, C. L., Norman, G. R. & Ali, S. H. Effect of Voice Recognition on Radiologist Reporting Time. *Can. Assoc. Radiol. J.* **59,** 203–209 (2008).

103. Singh, H. & Vij, M. S. Eight Recommendations for Policies for Communicating Abnormal Test Results. *Jt. Comm. J. Qual. Patient Saf.* **36,** 226–232 (2010).

104. Physician Quality Reporting System (PQRS) Overview. at <http://www.acr.org/Quality-Safety/Quality-Measurement/PQRS>

105. Seltzer, S. E. *et al.* Expediting the Turnaround of Radiology Reports: Use of Total Quality Management to Facilitate Radiologists' Report Signing. *AJR. Am. J. Roentgenol.* **162,** 775–781 (1994).

106. Holman, B. L. *et al.* Medical Impact of Unedited Preliminary Radiology Reports. *Radiology* **191,** 519–521 (1994).

107. Technology Adoption Life Cycle. at <https://en.wikipedia.org/wiki/Technology_adoption_lifecycle>

108. Bosmans, J. M. L. *et al.* Structured Reporting: If, Why, When, How-and at What Expense? Results of a Focus Group Meeting of Radiology Professionals from Eight Countries. *Insights Imaging* **3,** 295–302 (2012).

109. Kahn, C. E. *et al.* Toward Best Practices in Radiology Reporting. *Radiology* **252,** 852–856 (2009).

110. Good Practice for Radiological Reporting. Guidelines from the European Society of Radiology (ESR). *Insights Imaging* **2,** 93–96 (2011).

111. Sadigh, G., Loehfelm, T., Applegate, K. E. & Tridandapani, S. Evaluation of Near-Miss Wrong-Patient Events in Radiology Reports. *AJR. Am. J. Roentgenol.* **205,** 337–43 (2015).

112. Gale, M. E. & Gale, D. R. DICOM Modality Worklist: An Essential Component in a PACS Environment. *J. Digit. Imaging* **13,** 101–108 (2000).

113. Leslie, A., Jones, A. J. & Goddard, P. R. The Influence of Clinical Information on the Reporting of CT by Radiologists. *Br. J. Radiol.* **73,** 1052–1055 (2000).

114. Doubilet, P. & Herman, P. Interpretation of Radiographs: Effect of Clinical History. *Am. J. Roentgenol.* **137,** 1055–1058 (1981).

115. Berbaum, K. S., Franken, E. A. J., Dorfman, D. D. & Lueben, K. R. Influence of Clinical History on Perception of Abnormalities in Pediatric Radiographs. *Acad. Radiol.* **1,** 217–223 (1994).

116. Good, B. C. *et al.* Does Knowledge of the Clinical History Affect the Accuracy of Chest Radiograph Interpretation? *AJR. Am. J. Roentgenol.* **154,** 709–712 (1990).

117. Eldevik, O. P., Dugstad, G., Orrison, W. W. & Haughton, V. M. The Effect of Clinical Bias on the Interpretation of Myelography and Spinal Computed Tomography. *Radiology* **145,** 85–89 (1982).

118. Babcook, C. J., Norman, G. R. & Coblentz, C. L. Effect of Clinical History on the Interpretation of Chest Radiographs in Childhood Bronchiolitis. *Invest. Radiol.* **28,** 214–217 (1993).

119. Berbaum, K. S., Franken, E. A. J. & El-Khoury, G. Y. Impact of Clinical History on Radiographic Detection of Fractures: A Comparison of Radiologists and Orthopedists. *AJR. Am. J. Roentgenol.* **153,** 1221–1224 (1989).

120. Berbaum, K. S., Franken, E. A., Dorfman, D. D. & Barloon, T. J. Influence of Clinical History upon Detection of Nodules and Other Lesions. *Invest. Radiol.* **23,** 48–55 (1988).

121. Berbaum, K. S. & Franken, E. A. Commentary: Does Clinical History Affect Perception? *Acad. Radiol.* **13,** 402–403 (2006).

122. Mullins, M. E., Lev, M. H., Schellingerhout, D., Koroshetz, W. J. & Gonzalez, R. G. Influence of Availability of Clinical History on Detection of Early Stroke Using Unenhanced CT and Diffusion-Weighted MR Imaging. *AJR. Am. J. Roentgenol.* **179,** 223–8 (2002).

123. Schreiber, M. H. The Clinical History as a Factor in Roentgenogram Interpretation. *JAMA J. Am. Med. Assoc.* **185,** 399 (1963).

124. Loy, C. T. & Irwig, L. Accuracy of Diagnostic Tests Read with and without Clinical Information: A Systematic Review. *JAMA* **292,** 1602–1609 (2004).

125. Griscom, N. T. A Suggestion: Look at the Images First, Before You Read the History. *Radiology* **223,** 9–10 (2002).

126. Gaskin, C. EHR Driven Workflow for Diagnostic Radiologists - You Might Actually Want This. in *Annual Meeting of the Radiological*

Society of North America (Radiological Society of North America, 2013).

127. Boonn, W. W. & Langlotz, C. P. Radiologist Use of and Perceived Need for Patient Data Access. *J. Digit. Imaging* **22,** 357–362 (2009).

128. Fatahi, N., Krupic, F. & Hellström, M. Quality of Radiologists' Communication with Other Clinicians--As Experienced by Radiologists. *Patient Educ. Couns.* **98,** 722–727 (2015).

129. Abujudeh, H. H. *et al.* Computed tomography pulmonary angiography: an assessment of the radiology report. *Acad. Radiol.* **16,** 1309–15 (2009).

130. Revak, C. S. Dictation of Radiology Reports. *Am. J. Roentgenol.* **141,** 210 (1983).

131. ACR Practice Parameter for Communication of Diagnostic Imaging Findings. at <http://www.acr.org/~/media/ACR/Documents/PGTS/guidelines/Comm_Diag_Imaging.pdf>

132. Hunter, T. B. & Boyle, R. R. The Value of Reading the Previous Radiology Report. *Am. J. Roentgenol.* **150,** 697–698 (1988).

133. Aideyan, U. O., Berbaum, K. & Smith, W. L. Influence of Prior Radiologic Information on the Interpretation of Radiographic Examinations. *Acad. Radiol.* **2,** 205–208 (1995).

134. Doshi, A. M., Kiritsy, M. & Rosenkrantz, A. B. Strategies for Avoiding Recommendations for Additional Imaging Through a Comprehensive Comparison with Prior Studies. *J. Am. Coll. Radiol.* **12,** 657–63 (2015).

135. White, K., Berbaum, K. & Smith, W. L. The Role of Previous Radiographs and Reports in the Interpretation of Current Radiographs. *Invest. Radiol.* **29,** 263–265 (1994).

136. Deyo, R. A., McNiesh, L. M. & Cone, R. O. Observer Variability in the Interpretation of Lumbar Spine Radiographs. *Arthritis Rheum.* **28,** 1066–1070 (1985).

137. Elmore, J. G., Wells, C. K., Lee, C. H., Howard, D. H. & Feinstein, A. R. Variability in Radiologists' Interpretations of Mammograms. *N. Engl. J. Med.* **331,** 1493–1499 (1994).

138. Berlin, L. Comparing New Radiographs with Those Obtained Previously. *Am. J. Roentgenol.* **172**, 3–6 (1999).

139. Gunderman, R., Ambrosius, W. T. & Cohen, M. Radiology Reporting in an Academic Children's Hospital: What Referring Physicians Think. *Pediatr. Radiol.* **30**, 307–314 (2000).

140. ACR BI-RADS Atlas. at <http://www.acr.org/Quality-Safety/Resources/BIRADS>

141. Mitchell, D. G., Bruix, J., Sherman, M. & Sirlin, C. B. LI-RADS (Liver Imaging Reporting and Data System): Summary, Discussion, and Consensus of the LI-RADS Management Working Group and Future Directions. *Hepatology* **61**, 1056–1065 (2015).

142. Barentsz, J. O. *et al.* ESUR Prostate MR Guidelines 2012. *Eur. Radiol.* **22**, 746–57 (2012).

143. Head Injury Imaging Reporting and Data System. at <http://www.acr.org/Quality-Safety/Resources/HIRADS>

144. Pooler, B. D., Kim, D. H., Lam, V. P., Burnside, E. S. & Pickhardt, P. J. CT Colonography Reporting and Data System (C-RADS): Benchmark Values from a Clinical Screening Program. *AJR. Am. J. Roentgenol.* **202**, 1232–1237 (2014).

145. Orrison, W. W., Nord, T. E., Kinard, R. E. & Juhl, J. H. The Language of Certainty: Proper Terminology for the Ending of the Radiologic Report. *AJR. Am. J. Roentgenol.* **145**, 1093–1095 (1985).

146. Del Regato, J. Frances Henry Williams (1852-1896). 13–24 (1993). at <http://www.juanadelregatofoundation.org/Publications/BiographieshistoryObituariesEnglish/Radiological_Oncologists/Chapter 2.pdf>

147. Reiner, B. I. Strategies for Radiology Reporting and Communication : Part 2: Using Visual Imagery for Enhanced and Standardized Communication. *J. Digit. Imaging* **26**, 838–842 (2013).

148. Pendergrass, E. P. Francis Henry Williams, M.D. *Radiology* **60**, 737–738 (1953).

149. Williams, F. H. *The Roentgen Rays in Medicine and Surgery as an Aid in Diagnosis and as a Therapeutic Agent.* (The MacMillan Company, 1896).

150. Brolin, I. MEDELA: An Electronic Data-Processing System for Radiological Reporting. *Radiology* **103,** 249–255 (1972).

151. Bosmans, J. M. L. The Radiology Report: Communicating is a Profession, Writing a Passion. (Ghent University, 2011).

152. Nayak, L., Beaulieu, C. F., Rubin, D. L. & Lipson, J. A. A Picture is Worth a Thousand Words: Needs Assessment for Multimedia Radiology Reports in a Large Tertiary Care Medical Center. *Acad. Radiol.* **20,** 1577–1583 (2013).

153. Sadigh, G. *et al.* Traditional Text-Only Versus Multimedia-Enhanced Radiology Reporting: Referring Physicians' Perceptions of Value. *J. Am. Coll. Radiol.* **12,** 519–524 (2015).

154. Brown, L. R. A Tribute to Russell Daniel Carman. *Mayo Clin. Proc.* **70,** 1215–1217 (1995).

155. Carman, R. D. & Miller, A. *The Roentgen Diagnosis of Diseases of the Alimentary Canal.* (W. B. Saunders and Company, 1917).

156. Carman, R. D. The Making and Filing of Records in the Section on Roentgenology in the Mayo Clinic. *AJR. Am. J. Roentgenol.* **8,** 372–82 (1921).

157. Pendergrass, H. P. *et al.* An On-line Computer Facility for Systematized Input of Radiology Reports. *Radiology* **92,** 709–713 (1969).

158. Greenes, R. A., Barnett, G. O., Klein, S. W., Robbins, A. & Prior, R. E. Recording, Retrieval and Review of Medical Data by Physician-Computer Interaction. *N. Engl. J. Med.* **282,** 307–315 (1970).

159. Simon, M. *et al.* Computerized Radiology Reporting Using Coded Language. *Radiology* **113,** 343–349 (1974).

160. Templeton, A. W. *et al.* Radiate—Updated and Redesigned for Multiple Cathode-Ray Tube Terminals. *Radiology* **92,** 30–36 (1969).

161. Lehr, J. L., Lodwick, G. S., Nicholson, B. F. & Birznieks, F. B. Experience with MARS (Missouri Automated Radiology System). *Radiology* **106,** 289–294 (1973).

162. Wheeler, P. S., Simborg, D. W. & Gitlin, J. N. The Johns Hopkins Radiology Reporting System. *Radiology* **119,** 315–319 (1976).

163. Bluemke, D. A. & Eng, J. An Automated Radiology Reporting System that Uses HyperCard. *AJR. Am. J. Roentgenol.* **160,** 185–187 (1993).

164. Mani, R. L. & Jones, M. D. MSF: A Computer-Assisted Radiologic Reporting System. *Radiology* **108,** 587–596 (1973).

165. Mani, R. RAPORT Radiology System: Results of Clinical Trials. *Am. J. Roentgenol.* **127,** 811–816 (1976).

166. Irwin, G. A. L. & Tillitt, R. A Computer-assisted Radiological Reporting System. *Radiology* **118,** 239–331 (1976).

167. Sherman, R. S. An Automated System for Recording Reports of Chest Roentgenograms. *Am. J. Roentgenol.* **117,** 848–854 (1973).

168. Robbins, A. H., Vincent, M. E., Shaffer, K., Maietta, R. & Srinivasan, M. K. Radiology Reports: Assessment of a 5,000-Word Speech Recognizer. *Radiology* **167,** 853–855 (1988).

169. Morton, D. The History of Recording Technology. at <http://www.recording-history.org/HTML/dicta_biz1.php>

170. Blanding, M. Speechless. *Tufts Magazine* (2012). at <http://www.tufts.edu/alumni/magazine/fall2012/features/speechless.html>

171. Garfinkel, S. Enter the Dragon. *Technol. Rev.* **101,** 58–64 (1998).

172. Mobley, M, Qu, L, Sit, E, Wong, J. *Dragon Systems*. (1998). at <http://ocw.mit.edu/courses/electrical-engineering-and-computer-science/6-933j-the-structure-of-engineering-revolutions-fall-2001/projects/dragon.pdf>

173. Hoover, H. Annual Message to the Congress on the State of the Union. (1930). at <http://www.presidency.ucsb.edu/ws/?pid=22458>

174. Nuance CEO Confirms Siri Partnership with Apple. (2013). at <http://www.macrumors.com/2013/05/30/nuance-ceo-confirms-siri-partnership-with-apple/>

175. Sistrom, C. L. & Langlotz, C. P. A Framework for Improving Radiology Reporting. *J. Am. Coll. Radiol.* **2,** 159–167 (2005).

176. Langlotz, C. P. ACR BI-RADS for Breast Imaging Communication: A Roadmap for the Rest of Radiology. *J. Am. Coll. Radiol. JACR* **6**, 861–863 (2009).

177. Langlotz, C. P. Structured Radiology Reporting: Are We There Yet? *Radiology* **253**, 23–25 (2009).

178. Langlotz, C. Automatic Structuring of Radiology Reports: Harbinger of a Second Information Revolution in Radiology. *Radiology* **224**, 5–7 (2002).

179. Weiss, D. L. & Langlotz, C. P. Structured Reporting: Patient Care Enhancement or Productivity Nightmare? *Radiology* **249**, 739–747 (2008).

180. Englebart, D. C. *Study for the Development of Human Augmentation Techniques. Final Report for NASA Langley Research Center.* (1968). at <http://web.stanford.edu/dept/SUL/library/extra4/sloan/mousesite/Archive/Post68/FinalReport1968/study68developments.html>

181. Powell, D. K. & Silberzweig, J. E. State of Structured Reporting in Radiology, a Survey. *Acad. Radiol.* **22**, 226–233 (2015).

182. Rads Split on Use of Structured Reporting. at <http://www.diagnosticimaging.com/pacs-and-informatics/rads-split-use-structured-reporting>

183. Bell, D. S. & Greenes, R. A. Evaluation of UltraSTAR: Performance of a Collaborative Structured Data Entry System. *Proc. Annu. Symp. Comput. Appl. Med. Care* 216–222 (1994). at <http://www.ncbi.nlm.nih.gov/pmc/articles/PMC2247858/>

184. Kahn, C. E., Wang, K. & Bell, D. S. Structured Entry of Radiology Reports Using World Wide Web Technology. *RadioGraphics* **16**, 683–691 (1996).

185. Kanegaye, J. T., Cheng, J. C., McCaslin, R. I., Trocinski, D. & Silva, P. D. Improved Documentation of Wound Care with a Structured Encounter Form in the Pediatric Emergency Department. *Ambul. Pediatr. Off. J. Ambul. Pediatr. Assoc.* **5**, 253–257 (2005).

186. Silfen, E. Documentation and Coding of ED Patient Encounters: An Evaluation of the Accuracy of an Electronic Medical Record. *Am. J. Emerg. Med.* **24,** 664–678 (2006).

187. Eden, K. B. *et al.* Examining the Value of Electronic Health Records on Labor and Delivery. *Am. J. Obstet. Gynecol.* **199,** 307.e1–307.e9 (2008).

188. Tsai, J. & Bond, G. A Comparison of Electronic Records to Paper Records in Mental Health Centers. *Int. J. Qual. Heal. care J. Int. Soc. Qual. Heal. Care / ISQua* **20,** 136–143 (2008).

189. Soekhoe, J. K. *et al.* Computerized Endoscopic Reporting Is No more Time-consuming Than Reporting with Conventional Methods. *Eur. J. Intern. Med.* **18,** 321–325 (2007).

190. Clunie, D. A. *DICOM Structured Reporting.* (PixelMed Publishing, 2000).

191. Langlotz, C. P. Enhancing the Expressiveness of Structured Reporting Systems. *J. Digit. Imaging* **13,** 49–53 (2000).

192. Liu, D., Berman, G. D. & Gray, Richard N. The use of structured radiology reporting at a community hospital: A 4-year case study of more than 200,000 reports. *Appl. Radiol.* **32,** 23–26 (2003).

193. Langlotz, C. P. & Meininger, L. Enhancing the expressiveness and usability of structured image reporting systems. *Proc. AMIA Symp.* 467–471 (2000).

194. Langlotz, C. P. & Caldwell, S. A. The Completeness of Existing Lexicons for Representing Radiology Report Information. *J. Digit. Imaging* **15 Suppl 1,** 201–205 (2002).

195. Johnson, A. J., Chen, M. Y. M., Swan, J. S., Applegate, K. E. & Littenberg, B. Cohort Study of Structured Reporting Compared with Conventional Dictation. *Radiology* **253,** 74–80 (2009).

196. American College of Radiology. *Breast Image Reporting and Data System (BI-RADS) Atlas.* (American College of Radiology, 2003).

197. Stillman, A. E. *et al.* Structured Reporting: Coronary CT Angiography: A White Paper from the American College of Radiology and the North American Society for Cardiovascular Imaging. *J. Am. Coll. Radiol. JACR* **5,** 796–800 (2008).

198. Douglas, P. S. *et al.* ACCF/ACR/AHA/ASE/ASNC/HRS/NASCI/RSNA/SAIP/SCAI/SCCT/SCMR 2008 Health Policy Statement on Structured Reporting in Cardiovascular Imaging. *J. Am. Coll. Cardiol.* **53,** 76–90 (2009).

199. Gouveia-Oliveira, A. *et al.* Longitudinal Comparative Study on the Influence of Computers on Reporting of Clinical Data. *Endoscopy* **23,** 334–337 (2008).

200. Reiner, B. I., Knight, N. & Siegel, E. L. Radiology Reporting, Past, Present, and Future: The Radiologist's Perspective. *J. Am. Coll. Radiol.* **4,** 313–319 (2007).

201. Robinson, P. J. Radiology's Achilles' Heel: Error and Variation in the Interpretation of the Roentgen Image. *Br. J. Radiol.* **70,** 1085–1098 (1997).

202. Dunnick, N. R. & Langlotz, C. P. The Radiology Report of the Future: A Summary of the 2007 Intersociety Conference. *Journal of the American College of Radiology* **5,** 626–629 (2008).

203. Morgan, T. A., Heilbrun, M. E. & Kahn, C. E. Reporting Initiative of the Radiological Society of North America: Progress and New Directions. *Radiology* **273,** 642–645 (2014).

204. RSNA Informatics Reporting Initiative Metrics Page. (2015). at <http://radreport.org/metrics.php>

205. Kahn, C. E., Genereaux, B. & Langlotz, C. P. Conversion of Radiology Reporting Templates to the MRRT Standard. *J. Digit. Imaging* (2015). doi:10.1007/s10278-015-9787-3

206. Hickson, I, Berjon, R, Faulkner, S, Leithead, T, Navarra, ED, O'Connor, E, Pfeiffer, S. HTML5 A vocabulary and associated APIs for HTML and XHTML. (2014). at <http://www.w3.org/html/wg/drafts/html/CR/>

207. Tublin, M. E., Deible, C. R. & Shrestha, R. B. The Radiology Report Version 2.0. *J. Am. Coll. Radiol.* **12,** 217–219 (2015).

208. Chapman, W. W., Bridewell, W., Hanbury, P., Cooper, G. F. & Buchanan, B. G. A Simple Algorithm for Identifying Negated Findings and Diseases in Discharge Summaries. *J. Biomed. Inform.* **34,** 301–310 (2001).

209. Mehrabi, S. *et al.* DEEPEN: A Negation Detection System for Clinical Text Incorporating Dependency Relation into NegEx. *J. Biomed. Inform.* **54,** 213–219 (2015).

210. Danton, G. Radiology Reporting: Changes Worth Making are Never Easy. *Appl. Radiol.* 19–23 (2010).

211. FAA Recommends Pilots Spend Less Time Using Autopilot. at <https://www.nbaa.org/ops/safety/20130125-faa-recommends-pilots-spend-more-time-hand-flying-their-aircraft.php>

212. MacMahon, H. *et al.* Guidelines for Management of Small Pulmonary Nodules Detected on CT Scans: A Statement from the Fleischner Society. *Radiology* **237,** 395–400 (2005).

213. Naidich, D. P. *et al.* Recommendations for the Management of Subsolid Pulmonary Nodules Detected at CT: A Statement from the Fleischner Society. *Radiology* **266,** 304–317 (2013).

214. Itri, J. N., Redfern, R. O. & Scanlon, M. H. Using a Web-Based Application to Enhance Resident Training and Improve Performance On-call. *Acad. Radiol.* **17,** 917–920 (2010).

215. Itri, J. N., Kim, W. & Scanlon, M. H. Orion: A Web-based Application Designed to Monitor Resident and Fellow Performance On-call. *J. Digit. Imaging* **24,** 897–907 (2011).

216. Larson, D. B., Towbin, A. J., Pryor, R. M. & Donnelly, L. F. Improving Consistency In Radiology Reporting through the Use of Department-Wide Standardized Structured Reporting. *Radiology* **267,** 240–250 (2013).

217. Nunes, L. W. *et al.* Breast MR Imaging: Interpretation Model. *Radiology* **202,** 833–841 (1997).

218. Nunes, L. W., Schnall, M. D. & Orel, S. G. Update of Breast MR Imaging Architectural Interpretation Model. *Radiology* (2001). at <http://pubs.rsna.org/doi/abs/10.1148/radiology.219.2.r01ma44484>

219. Fatal airliner (14+ passengers) hull-loss accidents. at <http://aviation-safety.net/statistics/period/stats.php?cat=A1>

220. Burnside, E. S. *et al.* The ACR BI-RADS Experience: Learning from History. *J. Am. Coll. Radiol.* **6,** 851–860 (2009).

221. Berg, W. A. *et al.* Does Training in the Breast Imaging Reporting and Data System (BI-RADS) Improve Biopsy Recommendations or Feature Analysis Agreement with Experienced Breast Imagers at Mammography? *Radiology* **224,** 871–880 (2002).

222. Sickles, E. A. *et al.* Performance Benchmarks for Diagnostic Mammography. *Radiology* **235,** 775–790 (2005).

223. Rosenberg, R. D. *et al.* Performance Benchmarks for Screening Mammography. *Radiology* **241,** 55–66 (2006).

224. Caggiati, A. *et al.* Nomenclature of the Veins of the Lower Limbs: An International Interdisciplinary Consensus Statement. *J. Vasc. Surg.* **36,** 416–422 (2002).

225. Atkinson, R. P. *et al.* Reporting Terminology for Brain Arteriovenous Malformation Clinical and Radiographic Features for Use in Clinical Trials. *Stroke.* **32,** 1430–1442 (2001).

226. Fardon, D. F. *et al.* Lumbar disc nomenclature: version 2.0: Recommendations of the combined task forces of the North American Spine Society, the American Society of Spine Radiology and the American Society of Neuroradiology. *Spine J.* **14,** 2525–2545 (2014).

227. Lung CT Screening Reporting and Data System (Lung-RADS). at <http://www.acr.org/Quality-Safety/Resources/LungRADS>

228. SNOMED-CT: The Global Language of Healthcare. at <http://www.ihtsdo.org/snomed-ct>

229. Langlotz, C. P. RadLex: A New Method for Indexing Online Educational Materials. *Radiographics* **26,** 1595–1597 (2006).

230. RSNA Informatics: RadLex. at <http://radlex.org/>

231. RSNA Informatics: RadLex Playbook. at <http://playbook.radlex.org/>

232. American College of Radiology National Radiology Data Registry: Dose Index Registry. at <https://nrdr.acr.org/Portal/DIR/Main/page.aspx>

233. McDonald, C. J. *et al.* LOINC, a universal standard for identifying laboratory observations: a 5-year update. *Clin. Chem.* **49,** 624–33 (2003).

234. Boland, G. W. L. *et al.* Decision Support for Radiologist Report Recommendations. *J. Am. Coll. Radiol.* **8,** 819–823 (2011).

235. Langlotz, C. P. Fundamental measures of diagnostic examination performance: usefulness for clinical decision making and research. *Radiology* **228,** 3–9 (2003).

236. George Boole (1815 - 1864). at <http://www.kerryr.net/pioneers/boole.htm>

237. George Boole. at <https://en.wikipedia.org/wiki/George_Boole>

238. William Reville. The Greatness of George Boole. *Irish Times* (1996). at <http://undersci.ucc.ie/wp-content/uploads/sites/12/2014/11/George_Boole.pdf>

239. Hawking, S. *And God Created the Integers*. (Running Press Book Publishers, 2007).

240. Boole, G. The Laws of Thought, on Which Are Founded the Mathematical Theories of Logic and Probabilities. at <http://www.gutenberg.org/files/15114/15114-pdf.pdf>

241. Newell, HA, Simon, H. *Human Problem Solving*. (Prentice-Hall, 1972).

242. Bellhouse, D. R. The Reverend Thomas Bayes, FRS: A Biography to Celebrate the Tercentenary of His Birth. *Stat. Sci.* **19,** 3–43 (2004).

243. Price, M. B. and M. An Essay towards Solving a Problem in the Doctrine of Chances., By the Late Rev. Mr. Bayes, FRS Communicated By Mr. Price, in a Letter to John Canton AMFRS. *Phillosophical Trans.* **53,** 370–418 (1763).

244. An Essay towards solving a Problem in the Doctrine of Chances. at <http://en.wikipedia.org/wiki/An_Essay_towards_solving_a_Problem_in_the_Doctrine_of_Chances>

245. Pierre-Simon Laplace. at <https://en.wikipedia.org/wiki/Pierre-Simon_Laplace>

246. Laplace, P.-S. Memoir on the Probability of the Causes of Events. *Stat. Sci.* **1,** 364–378 (1986).

247. McGrayne, S. B. *The Theory That Would Not Die: How Bayes' Rule Cracked the Enigma Code, Hunted Down Russian Submarines, and*

Emerged Triumphant from Two Centuries of Controversy. (Yale University Press, 2012).

248. Stigler, S. M. Laplace's 1774 Memoir on Inverse Probability. *Stat. Sci.* **1,** 359–363 (1986).

249. Probability interpretations. at <https://en.wikipedia.org/wiki/Probability_interpretations>

250. Pearson, K. Laplace. *Biometrika* **21,** 202–216 (1929).

251. Karl Pearson. at <https://en.wikipedia.org/wiki/Karl_Pearson>

252. The Grammar of Science. at <https://en.wikipedia.org/wiki/The_Grammar_of_Science>

253. Burton, E. C., Troxclair, D. A. & Newman III, W. P. Autopsy Diagnoses of Malignant Neoplasms. *JAMA* **280,** 1245 (1998).

254. Hanley, J. A. & McNeil, B. J. The meaning and use of the area under a receiver operating characteristic (ROC) curve. *Radiology* **143,** 29–36 (1982).

255. Metz, C. E. Receiver Operating Characteristic Analysis: A Tool for the Quantitative Evaluation of Observer Performance and Imaging Systems. *J. Am. Coll. Radiol.* **3,** 413–422 (2006).

256. Brismar, J. Understanding receiver-operating-characteristic curves: a graphic approach. *AJR. Am. J. Roentgenol.* **157,** 1119–21 (1991).

257. Nunes, L. W. *et al.* Diagnostic performance characteristics of architectural features revealed by high spatial-resolution MR imaging of the breast. *AJR. Am. J. Roentgenol.* **169,** 409–415 (1997).

258. Pauker, S. G. & Kassirer, J. P. The threshold approach to clinical decision making. *N. Engl. J. Med.* **302,** 1109–17 (1980).

259. Ransohoff, D. F. & Feinstein, A. R. Problems of spectrum and bias in evaluating the efficacy of diagnostic tests. *N. Engl. J. Med.* **299,** 926–30 (1978).

260. Hillman, B. J. Outcomes research and cost-effectiveness analysis for diagnostic imaging. *Radiology* **193,** 307–10 (1994).

261. Sanger, E. L. In Memoriam: Lee B. Lusted, MD 1922-1994. *Radiology* **194,** 916 (1995).

262. Lusted, L. B. Signal detectability and medical decision-making. *Science* **171,** 1217–9 (1971).

263. Swets, J. Measuring the accuracy of diagnostic systems. *Science (80-.).* **240,** 1285–1293 (1988).

264. Hrung, J. M. *et al.* Cost-effectiveness of MR imaging and core-needle biopsy in the preoperative work-up of suspicious breast lesions. *Radiology* **213,** 39–49 (1999).

265. Filly, R. A. The 'lemon' sign: a clinical perspective. *Radiology* **167,** 573–5 (1988).

266. Black, W. C. & Armstrong, P. Communicating the significance of radiologic test results: the likelihood ratio. *AJR. Am. J. Roentgenol.* **147,** 1313–8 (1986).

267. Thornbury, J. R., Ornstein, D. K., Choyke, P. L., Langlotz, C. P. & Weinreb, J. C. Prostate cancer: what is the future role for imaging? *AJR. Am. J. Roentgenol.* **176,** 17–22 (2001).

268. Pascal. *Pensees.* (Guillaume Depres, 1670). at <https://en.wikisource.org/wiki/Pens%C3%A9es/IV>

269. Von Neumann, J, and Morgenstern, O. *Theory of Games and Economic Behavior.* (Princeton University Press, 1944).

270. Oshima Lee, E. & Emanuel, E. J. Shared decision making to improve care and reduce costs. *N. Engl. J. Med.* **368,** 6–8 (2013).

271. Plante, D. A., Kassirer, J. P., Zarin, D. A. & Pauker, S. G. Clinical decision consultation service. *Am. J. Med.* **80,** 1169–76 (1986).

272. Gorry, G. A. & Barnett, G. O. Experience with a model of sequential diagnosis. *Comput. Biomed. Res.* **1,** 490–507 (1968).

273. Schwartz, W. B. Sounding board. Decision Analysis: a look at the chief complaints. *N. Engl. J. Med.* **300,** 556–9 (1979).

274. Gardner, H. *The Mind's New Science: A History Of The Cognitive Revolution.* (Basic Books, 2008).

275. Gladwell, M. *David and Goliath.* (Little Brown and Company, 2013).

276. Tversky, A. & Kahneman, D. Judgment under Uncertainty: Heuristics and Biases. *Science* **185,** 1124–31 (1974).

277. Crowley, R. S. *et al.* Automated detection of heuristics and biases among pathologists in a computer-based system. *Adv. Health Sci. Educ. Theory Pract.* **18,** 343–63 (2013).

278. Wallsten, T. S. Physician and medical student bias in evaluating diagnostic information. *Med. Decis. Making* **1,** 145–64 (1981).

279. Bornstein, B. H. & Emler, A. C. Rationality in medical decision making: a review of the literature on doctors' decision-making biases. *J. Eval. Clin. Pract.* **7,** 97–107 (2001).

280. Elstein, A. S. Evidence base of clinical diagnosis: Clinical problem solving and diagnostic decision making: selective review of the cognitive literature. *BMJ* **324,** 729–732 (2002).

281. Kahneman, D, Slovic, P, Tversky, A. *Judgment Under Uncertainty: Heuristics and Biases.* (Cambridge University Press, 1982).

282. Schwartz, L. M., Woloshin, S. & Welch, H. G. Not so silver lining. *Arch. Intern. Med.* **171,** 489–90 (2011).

283. Pravettoni, G., Gorini, A., Bonanni, B. & Veronesi, U. The role of heuristics and biases in cancer-related decisions. *Ecancermedicalscience* **7,** ed26 (2013).

284. Medical students' disease. at <http://en.wikipedia.org/wiki/Medical_students%27_disease>

285. McNeil, B. J., Pauker, S. G., Sox, H. C. & Tversky, A. On the elicitation of preferences for alternative therapies. *N. Engl. J. Med.* **306,** 1259–62 (1982).

286. Kassirer, J. P. & Pauker, S. G. The toss-up. *N. Engl. J. Med.* **305,** 1467–9 (1981).

287. Muroff, L. R. Culture shift: an imperative for future survival. *J. Am. Coll. Radiol.* **10,** 93–8 (2013).

288. Zafar, H. M., Mills, A. M., Khorasani, R. & Langlotz, C. P. Clinical decision support for imaging in the era of the patient protection and affordable care act. *JACR J. Am. Coll. Radiol.* **9,** 907–918.e5 (2012).

289. Allen, B. Five reasons radiologists should embrace clinical decision support for diagnostic imaging. *J. Am. Coll. Radiol.* **11,** 533–4 (2014).

290. Duszak, R. & Berlin, J. W. Utilization management in radiology, part 1: rationale, history, and current status. *J. Am. Coll. Radiol.* **9,** 694–9 (2012).

291. Boland, G. W., Duszak, R. & Kalra, M. Protocol design and optimization. *J. Am. Coll. Radiol.* **11,** 440–1 (2014).

292. Zimmerman, S. L., Kim, W. & Boonn, W. W. Automated structured reporting of imaging findings using the AIM standard and XML. *Radiographics* **31,** 881–7 (2011).

293. Paulett, J. M. & Langlotz, C. P. Improving language models for radiology speech recognition. *J. Biomed. Inform.* **42,** 53–58 (2009).

294. Lee, Y. H., Yang, J. & Suh, J.-S. Detection and Correction of Laterality Errors in Radiology Reports. *J. Digit. Imaging* **28,** 412–6 (2015).

295. Dreyer, K. J. *et al.* Application of recently developed computer algorithm for automatic classification of unstructured radiology reports: validation study. *Radiology* **234,** 323–9 (2005).

296. Hripcsak, G., Austin, J. H. M., Alderson, P. O. & Friedman, C. Use of natural language processing to translate clinical information from a database of 889,921 chest radiographic reports. *Radiology* **224,** 157–63 (2002).

297. Do, B. H., Wu, A. S., Maley, J. & Biswal, S. Automatic retrieval of bone fracture knowledge using natural language processing. *J. Digit. Imaging* **26,** 709–13 (2013).

298. Budovec, J. J., Lam, C. A. & Kahn, C. E. Radiology gamuts ontology: differential diagnosis for the Semantic Web. *Radiographics* **34,** 254–64 (2014).

299. Burnside, E. S. *et al.* Bayesian Network to Predict Breast Cancer Risk of Mammographic Microcalcifications and Reduce Number of Benign Biopsy Results: Initial Experience 1. *Radiology* **240,** 666–673 (2006).

300. Bouzghar, G. *et al.* Bayesian Probability of Malignancy With BI-RADS Sonographic Features. *J. Ultrasound Med.* **33,** 641–648 (2014).

301. Soardi, G. A., Perandini, S., Motton, M. & Montemezzi, S. Assessing probability of malignancy in solid solitary pulmonary nodules with a new Bayesian calculator: improving diagnostic accuracy by means of expanded and updated features. *Eur. Radiol.* **25,** 155–62 (2015).

302. Benndorf, M. *et al.* Development of an online, publicly accessible naive Bayesian decision support tool for mammographic mass lesions based on the American College of Radiology (ACR) BI-RADS lexicon. *Eur. Radiol.* **25,** 1768–75 (2015).

303. Schell, M. J. *et al.* Evidence-based target recall rates for screening mammography. *Radiology* **243,** 681–9 (2007).

304. Langer, S. G. *et al.* The RSNA Image Sharing Network. *J. Digit. Imaging* **28,** 53–61 (2015).

305. Kaushal, R., Shojania, K. G. & Bates, D. W. Effects of computerized physician order entry and clinical decision support systems on medication safety: a systematic review. *Arch. Intern. Med.* **163,** 1409–16 (2003).

306. Jollis, J. G. *et al.* Discordance of databases designed for claims payment versus clinical information systems. Implications for outcomes research. *Ann. Intern. Med.* **119,** 844–50 (1993).

307. Reiner, B. & Siegel, E. Radiology reporting: returning to our image-centric roots. *AJR. Am. J. Roentgenol.* **187,** 1151–5 (2006).

308. Friedman, C., Alderson, P. O., Austin, J. H. M., Cimino, J. J. & Johnson, S. B. A general natural-language text processor for clinical radiology. *J. Am. Med. Informatics Assoc.* **1,** 161–174 (1994).

309. Friedman, C., Rindflesch, T. C. & Corn, M. Natural language processing: State of the art and prospects for significant progress, a workshop sponsored by the National Library of Medicine. *J. Biomed. Inform.* **46,** 765–773 (2013).

310. Knirsch, C. A., Jain, N. L., Pablos-Mendez, A., Friedman, C. & Hripcsak, G. Respiratory isolation of tuberculosis patients using clinical guidelines and an automated clinical decision support system. *Infect. Control Hosp. Epidemiol.* **19,** 94–100 (1998).

311. Taira, R. K. & Soderland, S. G. A statistical natural language processor for medical reports. *Proc. AMIA Symp.* 970–4 (1999). at <http://www.pubmedcentral.nih.gov/articlerender.fcgi?artid=2232848&tool=pmcentrez&rendertype=abstract>

312. Hripcsak, G, Kuperman, GJ, Friedman, C. Extracting findings from narrative reports: Software transferability and sources of physician disagreement. *Meth Info Med* **37,** 1–7 (1998).

313. Elkins, J. S., Friedman, C., Boden-Albala, B., Sacco, R. L. & Hripcsak, G. Coding neuroradiology reports for the Northern Manhattan Stroke Study: a comparison of natural language processing and manual review. *Comput. Biomed. Res.* **33,** 1–10 (2000).

314. Wang, S. & Summers, R. M. Machine learning and radiology. *Med. Image Anal.* **16,** 933–51 (2012).

315. Hassanpour, S. & Langlotz, C. P. Information extraction from multi-institutional radiology reports. *Artif. Intell. Med.* (2015). doi:10.1016/j.artmed.2015.09.007

316. Larson, P. A., Berland, L. L., Griffith, B., Kahn, C. E. & Liebscher, L. A. Actionable findings and the role of IT support: report of the ACR Actionable Reporting Work Group. *J. Am. Coll. Radiol.* **11,** 552–8 (2014).

317. Khorasani, R. Optimizing communication of critical test results. *J. Am. Coll. Radiol.* **6,** 721–3 (2009).

318. Johnson, A. J., Easterling, D., Nelson, R., Chen, M. Y. & Frankel, R. M. Access to radiologic reports via a patient portal: clinical simulations to investigate patient preferences. *J. Am. Coll. Radiol.* **9,** 256–63 (2012).

Index

Disclosures

I have received financial or in-kind research support from the following companies, government agencies, and professional organizations: the National Institute for Biomedical Imaging and Bioengineering (NIBIB), the Center for Medicare and Medicaid Services (CMS), the National Cancer Institute (NCI), the Radiological Society of North America (RSNA), the Society for Imaging Informatics in Medicine (SIIM), the Association of University Radiologists, GE Healthcare, Siemens Medical Systems, Medicalis, and Radimetrics.

I currently serve on the advisory boards of two companies: Elsevier, Inc. (Physician Advisory Board), and Activate Networks, Inc. (Advisory Board)

I have been a founder of three radiology-related businesses. I founded Access Radiology, a vendor of image solutions (PACS), in 1992. I no longer have a financial interest in that business, which is now a part of Merge Technologies, Inc., recently acquired by IBM.

I founded eDictation, Inc., a developer of structured reporting software in 1998 and served as its president and CEO. eDictation ceased operations in 2004.

I am a founder of Montage Healthcare, Inc., an enterprise search and analytics vendor for radiology practices, established in 2010. I remain an investor and shareholder and serve on its board of directors.

Acknowledgments

I am indebted to Jan Bosmans, Chuck Kahn, Ram Chadalavada, Harry Jha, and David Larson for providing many insightful comments on an early draft of this book.

Sue Harmon was an indispensable editor, reigning in my wilder impulses, and enforcing consistency. Any faults in the final manuscript are my own.

Special gratitude goes out to David Weiss and Chris Sistrom for allowing me to adapt our collaborative work in portions of this book. Nisha Mehta helped me organize my speech bloopers.

Great thanks are due to the radiology residents, fellows, students, and post-doctoral scholars with whom I have worked at the University of Pennsylvania and Stanford University. Your questions and curiosity made me a better radiologist and catalyzed my interest in the radiology report.

I am fortunate to have learned from outstanding mentors during my career, including Richard Yonker, Ted Shortliffe, Sandy Schwartz, Hal Kundel, and Michael Bleshman.

I am particularly grateful to work with the Montage team and all my other young colleagues, who keep me on my toes.

And finally, my thanks go to the RSNA, ARRS, ACR, Elsevier, the Clendening History of Medicine Library at the University of Kansas, and the New York Academy of Medicine Library for providing the rights to historical material in this book.

About the Author

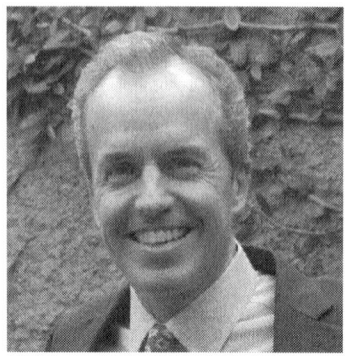

Curtis P. Langlotz, MD, PhD, serves as Professor of Radiology and Biomedical Informatics at Stanford University and as a Medical Informatics Director for Stanford Health Care. Over the past decade, Dr. Langlotz has led many national and international efforts to improve the quality of radiology reports, including the RadLex terminology standard, the RadLex Playbook of radiology exam codes, and the report template library of the Radiological Society of North America (RSNA). His research is focused on improving the accuracy and consistency of radiology communication through real-time decision support systems and other information technologies. His biomedical informatics laboratory develops novel machine learning and natural language processing algorithms that provide intelligent assistance to radiologists, clinicians, patients, and other consumers of the radiology report.

Dr. Langlotz is a founder and former president of the Radiology Alliance for Health Services Research (RAHSR), a former chair of the Society for Imaging Informatics in Medicine (SIIM), and a former board member of the Association of University Radiologists (AUR). He is a recipient of the Lee B. Lusted Prize from the Society of Medical Decision Making. He currently serves as a board member of the American Medical Informatics Association and as an informatics advisor to the RSNA. He has been elected a fellow of the American College of Medical Informatics and of the College of SIIM Fellows.

Raised in St. Paul, Minnesota, Dr. Langlotz received his undergraduate degree in Human Biology, masters in Computer Science, MD in Medicine, and PhD in Medical Information Science, all from Stanford University. He trained in radiology at the University of Pennsylvania, and served on the faculty there for 20 years. He lives in Menlo Park, California.

Printed in Great Britain
by Amazon